AUDIOLOGY AND HEARING RESEARCH ADVANCES

ADVANCES IN
AUDIOLOGY RESEARCH

AUDIOLOGY AND
HEARING RESEARCH ADVANCES

Additional books and e-books in this series can be found on Nova's website under the Series tab.

AUDIOLOGY AND HEARING RESEARCH ADVANCES

ADVANCES IN AUDIOLOGY RESEARCH

VICTOR M. KRISTENSEN
EDITOR

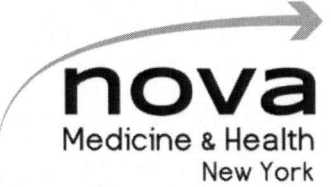

Copyright © 2019 by Nova Science Publishers, Inc.

All rights reserved. No part of this book may be reproduced, stored in a retrieval system or transmitted in any form or by any means: electronic, electrostatic, magnetic, tape, mechanical photocopying, recording or otherwise without the written permission of the Publisher.

We have partnered with Copyright Clearance Center to make it easy for you to obtain permissions to reuse content from this publication. Simply navigate to this **publication's** page on Nova's website and locate the "Get Permission" button below the title description. This button is linked directly to the title's permission page on copyright.com. Alternatively, you can visit copyright.com and search by title, ISBN, or ISSN.

For further questions about using the service on copyright.com, please contact:
Copyright Clearance Center
Phone: +1-(978) 750-8400   Fax: +1-(978) 750-4470   E-mail: info@copyright.com

NOTICE TO THE READER

The Publisher has taken reasonable care in the preparation of this book, but makes no expressed or implied warranty of any kind and assumes no responsibility for any errors or omissions. No liability is assumed for incidental or consequential damages in connection with or arising out of information contained in this book. The Publisher shall not be liable for any special, consequential, or exemplary damages resulting, in whole or in part, from the **readers'** use of, or reliance upon, this material. Any parts of this book based on government reports are so indicated and copyright is claimed for those parts to the extent applicable to compilations of such works.

Independent verification should be sought for any data, advice or recommendations contained in this book. In addition, no responsibility is assumed by the Publisher for any injury and/or damage to persons or property arising from any methods, products, instructions, ideas or otherwise contained in this publication.

This publication is designed to provide accurate and authoritative information with regard to the subject matter covered herein. It is sold with the clear understanding that the Publisher is not engaged in rendering legal or any other professional services. If legal or any other expert assistance is required, the services of a competent person should be sought. FROM A DECLARATION OF PARTICIPANTS JOINTLY ADOPTED BY A COMMITTEE OF THE AMERICAN BAR ASSOCIATION AND A COMMITTEE OF PUBLISHERS.

Additional color graphics may be available in the e-book version of this book.

Library of Congress Cataloging-in-Publication Data

ISBN: 978-1-53615-260-9

Published by Nova Science Publishers, Inc. † New York

CONTENTS

Preface		**vii**
Chapter 1	Genetics of Hearing Loss: Testing Methodologies and Counseling of Audiology Patients and Their Families *Danielle Donovan Mercer*	**1**
Chapter 2	Audiological and Surgical Outcome after Cochlear Implant Revision Surgery *Mohamed Salah Elgandy, Marlan R. Hansen and Richard S. Tyler*	**75**
Chapter 3	The Relationship between Self-Reported Restriction in Social Participation, Self-Reported Satisfaction/Benefit and the Time of Use of Hearing Aids *João Paulo N. A. Santos, Nathany L. Ruschel, Camila Z. Neves and Adriane R. Teixeira*	**99**

Chapter 4	Posturology: The Scientific Investigation of Postural Disorders *Giuseppe Messina, Valerio Giustino,* *Francesco Dispenza, Francesco Galletti,* *Angelo Iovane, Serena Rizzo* *and Francesco Martines*	117
Chapter 5	The Influence of Otovestibular System on Body Posture *Francesco Martines, Valerio Giustino,* *Francesco Dispenza, Francesco Galletti,* *Angelo Iovane, Serena Rizzo* *and Giuseppe Messina*	129
Chapter 6	Auditory Brainstem Response and Frequency Following Response in Patients with Sickle Cell Disease *Adriana L. Silveira, Adriane R. Teixeira,* *Christina M. Bittar, João Ricardo Friedrisch,* *Daniela P. Dall'Igna* *and Sergio S. Menna Barreto*	141
Index		159
Related Nova Publications		167

PREFACE

Genes causing hearing loss display various modes of inheritance, with autosomal recessive being the most common. With so many cases of hearing loss having a genetic etiology, audiologists are certain to encounter these patients on a fairly regular basis. Audiologists who possess basic knowledge about genetics are better equipped to recognize when a genetics referral is warranted, thereby enhancing patient care. In this chapter, it is determined that a genetics evaluation can yield valuable information for patients and their families, such as prognosis, estimates of recurrence risks, and diagnosis of other family members.

The second chapter will review causes of revision surgery, how to diagnose cases of failed cochlear implants and will discuss surgical and audiological outcome of revision cochlear implant surgeries, Speech recognition ability with a replacement cochlear implant may significantly increase or decrease from that with the original implant. Experienced cochlear implant patients facing reimplantation must be counseled regarding the possibility of differences in sound quality and speech recognition performance with their replacement device.

The purpose of the following chapter is to correlate the results obtained through questionnaires concerning self-reported restriction in social participation and patient satisfaction / benefit with objective time assessment of device use. This is a descriptive, cross-sectional study sample composed of and elderly and non-elderly adults of both sexes diagnosed with hearing loss and approved as candidates for hearing aid fitting at a university hospital.

The goal of chapter four is to understand the main features of human posture and how it is possible to analyze it.

The aim of this chapter is to investigate the influence of hearing loss and vestibular disorders on body posture.

The objective of the concluding chapter was to analyze the auditory brainstem response (ABR) and frequency following response (FFR) in patients diagnosed with Sickle Cell Disease (SCD) who were referred to the outpatient hemoglobinopathy clinic at a public hospital in southern Brazil.

Chapter 1 - Genes causing hearing loss display various modes of inheritance, with autosomal recessive being the most common. With so many cases of hearing loss having a genetic etiology, audiologists are certain to encounter these patients on a fairly regular basis. Audiologists who possess basic knowledge about genetics are better equipped to recognize when a genetics referral is warranted, thereby enhancing patient care. In this chapter, it is determined that a genetics evaluation can yield valuable information for patients and their families, such as prognosis, estimates of recurrence risks, and diagnosis of other family members. The second chapter will review causes of revision surgery, how to diagnose cases of failed cochlear implants and will discuss surgical and audiological outcome of revision cochlear implant surgeries, Speech recognition ability with a replacement cochlear implant may significantly increase or decrease from that with the original implant. Experienced cochlear implant patients facing reimplantation must be counseled regarding the possibility of differences in sound quality and speech recognition performance with their replacement device. The purpose of the following chapter is to correlate the results obtained through questionnaires concerning self-reported restriction in social participation and patient satisfaction / benefit with objective time assessment of device use. This is a descriptive, cross-sectional study sample composed of and elderly and non-elderly adults of both sexes diagnosed with hearing loss and approved as candidates for hearing aid fitting at a university hospital. The goal of chapter four is to understand the main features of human posture and how it is possible to analyze it. The aim of this chapter is to investigate the influence of hearing loss and vestibular disorders on body posture. The objective of the concluding chapter was to analyze the auditory brainstem response (ABR) and frequency following response (FFR) in patients diagnosed with Sickle Cell Disease (SCD) who were referred to the outpatient hemoglobinopathy clinic at a public hospital in southern Brazil.

Chapter 2 - Cochlear implantation is now widely accepted as a safe and effective treatment for children and adults with profound deafness. As with all electronic devices, a cochlear implant (CI) is susceptible to breakdown or failure. Although the CI reliability rate is now very high, the continually increasing population of implant recipients will result in the continued need for revision surgeries. The first report of a CI revision surgery occurred in 1985, by Hochmair-Desoyer and Burian. Since then, several reports have addressed the safety of this procedure, including the preservation or increase of speech per ception performance, although there have also been reports of decreases in electrode activation, decreased speech per ception and intra cochlear trauma, suggesting that cochlear reimplantation may have negative functional consequences in some patients, requiring careful consideration of the expected indications and benefits. This paper will review causes of revision surgery, how to diagnose cases of failed CI and will discuss surgical and audiological outcome of revision CI surgeries, Speech recognition ability with a replacement CI may significantly increase or decrease from that with the original implant. Experienced CI patients facing reimplantation must be counseled regarding the possibility of differences in sound quality and speech recognition performance with their replacement device.

Chapter 3 - To correlate the results obtained through questionnaires concerning self-reported restriction in social participation and patient satisfaction/benefit with objective time assessment of device use. This is a descriptive, cross-sectional study sample composed of and elderly and non-elderly adults of both sexes diagnosed with hearing loss and approved as candidates for hearing aid fitting at a university hospital. Subjects answered questionnaires that measure restriction in social participation restriction and user satisfaction/benefit, namely the Hearing Handicap Inventory for Adults (HHIA) for non-elderly adult patients; the Hearing Handicap Inventory for the Elderly Screening Version (HHIE-S), for elderly patients, and the International Outcome Inventory for Hearing Aids (IOI-HA) for both age groups. Average daily usage time of the devices was verified objectively through datalogging. A total of 49 users elderly and non-elderly of both sexes participated in the study. Self-reported hearing aid times of use were compared with those measured by datalogging. There was overestimation on the part of patients when reporting hearing aid use, which was verified when compared with software data. There was no significant correlation between questionnaire scores and the datalogged time of use. There was a negative correlation between the HHIE-S and IOI-HA questionnaires, and a positive correlation between the variable of age and the IOI-HA questionnaire, as well as another positive correlation between the variable of sex and the HHIA questionnaire. No relation was found between datalogged time of use and self-reported restriction in social participation or hearing aid user satisfaction/benefit.

Chapter 4 - To correlate the results obtained through questionnaires concerning self-reported restriction in social participation and patient satisfaction/benefit with objective time assessment of device use. This is a descriptive, cross-sectional study sample composed of and elderly and non-elderly adults of both sexes diagnosed with hearing loss and approved as candidates for hearing aid fitting at a university hospital. Subjects answered questionnaires that measure restriction in social participation restriction and user satisfaction/benefit, namely the Hearing Handicap Inventory for Adults (HHIA) for non-elderly adult patients; the Hearing Handicap Inventory for the Elderly Screening Version (HHIE-S), for elderly patients, and the International Outcome Inventory for Hearing Aids (IOI-HA) for both age groups. Average daily usage time of the devices was verified objectively through datalogging. A total of 49 users elderly and non-elderly of both sexes participated in the study. Self-reported hearing aid times of use were compared with those measured by datalogging. There was overestimation on the part of patients when reporting hearing aid use, which was verified when compared with software data. There was no significant correlation between questionnaire scores and the datalogged time of use. There was a negative correlation between the HHIE-S and IOI-HA questionnaires, and a positive correlation between the variable of age and the IOI-HA questionnaire, as well as another positive correlation between the variable of sex and the HHIA questionnaire. No relation was found between datalogged time of use and self-reported restriction in social participation or hearing aid user satisfaction/benefit.

Chapter 5 - It is well-known that body posture is controlled by an integration, at the level of the central nervous system, of afferences coming from various organs that influences the tonic postural system responsible for the alignment of the skeletal body segment of the human body, for balance and for postural control. Many studies have shown that the auditory and the vestibular systems contribute significantly to posture. The scientific literature reported that patients suffering from hearing impairment or vestibular disorders may be affected by loss of balance or inability to maintain postural control. Furthermore, many researchers have demonstrated a significant correlation between hearing loss and the risk of falling. Non-physiological sensory information from the otovestibular system negatively interferes on posture inducing asymmetrical muscular tensions that determines postural disorders. In these patients, a postural sway analysis, using a stabilometric platform, and a gait analysis, through a dynamic baropodometric test, can be considered in order to measure their ability to maintain static and dynamic balance and to examine their potential improvement after an otovestibular rehabilitation. The aim of this work is to investigate the influence of hearing loss and vestibular disorders on body posture.

Chapter 6 - The aim of this study was to analyze the auditory brainstem response (ABR) and frequency following response (FFR) in patients diagnosed with Sickle Cell Disease (SCD) who were referred to the outpatient hemoglobinopathy clinic at a public hospital in southern Brazil. Fifty-four individuals aged between 6 and 24 years [mean age ± SD (years), 14.1 ± 4.6] were evaluated. Pure tone audiometry, high frequency tonal audiometry, tympanometry, and transient evoked otoacoustic emission for determination of peripheral normality were performed; the overall results indicted normal auditory thresholds in all individuals. Subsequently, electrophysiological evaluations including ABR and FFR were performed; the analysis of the ABR responses revealed an alteration in 88.9% of the individuals and that of FFR in 98.1%. The achievement of auditory thresholds within the normal range and presence of otoacoustic emissions enabled but did not guarantee excellence in the auditory pathway of the evaluated individuals.

In: Advances in Audiology Research
Editor: Victor M. Kristensen

ISBN: 978-1-53615-260-9
© 2019 Nova Science Publishers, Inc.

Chapter 1

GENETICS OF HEARING LOSS: TESTING METHODOLOGIES AND COUNSELING OF AUDIOLOGY PATIENTS AND THEIR FAMILIES

Danielle Donovan Mercer[*]
State of Louisiana Early Hearing Detection and Intervention Program,
New Orleans, LA, US

ABSTRACT

Approximately 2 to 3 per 1,000 newborns are diagnosed with permanent hearing loss. It is estimated that 75 to 80% of these cases are due to a genetic etiology. Genetic hearing loss can be syndromic, meaning other clinical features are present along with the hearing loss; or nonsyndromic, meaning hearing loss occurs in isolation. More than 400 genes have been reported to contribute to hearing loss and more than 100 genes have been reported to cause nonsyndromic hearing loss. Genes

---

[*] Corresponding Author's E-mail: Danielle.Mercer@la.gov (AuD, MS, CG(ASCP)[CM]).

causing hearing loss display various modes of inheritance, with autosomal recessive being the most common. With so many cases of hearing loss having a genetic etiology, audiologists are certain to encounter these patients on a fairly regular basis. Audiologists who possess basic knowledge about genetics are better equipped to recognize when a genetics referral is warranted, thereby enhancing patient care. A genetics evaluation can yield valuable information for patients and their families, such as prognosis, estimates of recurrence risks, and diagnosis of other family members. A variety of testing methodologies are available, and are chosen based on such considerations as clinical presentation, cost, analysis time, laboratory availability, previous testing performed, and likelihood of a positive result, among others. As technologies for genetic testing advance, sequencing techniques such as whole exome sequencing, genomic sequencing, and targeted sequencing are becoming more affordable, allowing for more patients to receive a diagnosis than was previously possible.

Keywords: genetics, hearing loss, deafness, audiology, hearing loss counseling, sequencing, syndromic hearing loss, nonsyndromic hearing loss, genetic testing

1. INTRODUCTION

Approximately 2 to 3 per 1,000 newborns will be diagnosed with permanent hearing loss [1], making it one of the most common birth conditions. When factoring in delayed-onset and minimal hearing losses, prevalence increases to 20% in adolescence [2]. Historically, 50% of these cases have been attributed to genetic causes and 50% to environmental causes [3, 4]. However, estimates in recent years have suggested that the true proportion of permanent childhood hearing loss cases attributable to genetics in developed countries is closer to 80% [5]. This perceived increase in genetic hearing loss is likely due to a decrease in cases caused by infections, such as rubella. Prenatal rubella infection, a common cause of deafness in the 1960s and prior, has largely been eradicated in developed countries through vaccination [6]. Thus, the proportion of permanent hearing loss cases with a genetic etiology has increased. In addition, it is unknown how many genetic causes are undiagnosed. New epidemiological studies are needed to more accurately characterize the etiology of permanent childhood hearing loss.

The human genome contains approximately 20,000 genes [7]. These genes code for proteins which carry out all of the functions necessary for life. More than 400 genes have been reported to contribute to hearing loss [8] and more than 100 genes have been reported to cause hearing loss in isolation [9]. For a better understanding of genes, it is important to discuss what makes up genes: DNA.

2. DNA PROVIDES THE GENETIC CODE

2.1. Structure of DNA

DNA (deoxyribonucleic acid) is a nucleic acid. Nucleic acids are one of the four biological macromolecules essential for life, along with carbohydrates, proteins, and lipids. The structure of DNA was first described in 1953 by James Watson and Francis Crick, whose predictions were assisted by radiographs taken by Rosalind Franklin and suggested by Maurice Wilkins. Despite the complexity of functions required of the genetic code by humans and other species alike, the structure of DNA was found to exhibit surprising simplicity.

DNA is made up of nitrogen-containing bases called nucleotides bound to a sugar-phosphate backbone. The sugar is deoxyribose, a 5-carbon sugar. While the sugar-phosphate backbone remains constant, the nucleotides do not. There are four different nitrogenous bases in DNA: adenine, guanine, cytosine, and thymine, commonly abbreviated as A, G, C, and T, respectively. A and G are classified as purines (double-ringed structures) while C and T are classified as pyrimidines (single-ringed structures). DNA is structured as two chains which form a double helix shape (Figure 1). The two strands are connected via hydrogen bonds between bases on each strand. The bases form bonds in predictable fashion: A always bonds with T, and G always bonds with C. The two strands are thus complementary. These bases make up the genetic code.

Genes are transcribed into mRNA (messenger RNA), which is in turn translated into proteins.

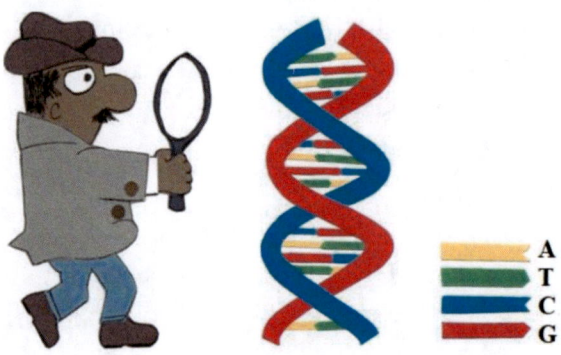

Figure 1. DNA structure. DNA is structured into a double helix with 4 nucleic acid bases: adenine (A), guanine (G), cytosine (C), and thymine (T). Adenine always pairs with thymine while guanine always pairs with cytosine. AT pairs are connected with two hydrogen bonds while GC pairs are connected with three hydrogen bonds.

2.2. DNA Is Packaged into Chromosomes

The roughly 3 billion base pairs of DNA that make up the human genome must be packaged into cells [10]. To accomplish this, DNA utilizes several mechanisms of compaction, which includes involvement of various proteins such as histones [11]. The human genome is arranged into 46 chromosomes. When the chromosomes are at maximal condensation, they can be stained and analyzed microscopically (see Section 6.1.1). The chromosomes are located in the nucleus of the cell. Most cells of the human body have 46 chromosomes packaged in the nucleus. Notable exceptions are the gametes (egg and sperm cells), which contain 23 chromosomes, and mature red blood cells, which do not have a nucleus. Somatic cells (cells that are not gametes) divide through a process known as mitosis, while gametes divide via meiosis. Mitosis and meiosis are similar processes, but meiosis involves two cell divisions as compared to one cell division in mitosis. Both processes precede with DNA replication (doubling). Mitosis follows with a division into two daughter cells each with the same amount of DNA as the parent cell. Meiosis follows with two cell divisions resulting in four daughter cells with half the amount of DNA as the parent cell.

2.3. Chromosomes Come in Pairs

The 46 chromosomes that contain the human genome consist of 23 pairs. One pair is inherited from a person's mother and one pair is inherited from the father. Egg and sperm cells contain 23 chromosomes each, creating a zygote with 46 chromosomes when they come together. The chromosomes are designated as either autosomes or sex chromosomes. The sex chromosomes are X and Y, and they determine sex. Females possess an XX sex chromosome complement, while males possess an XY chromosome complement. When passing on a sex chromosome to a child, females can only pass on an X chromosome.

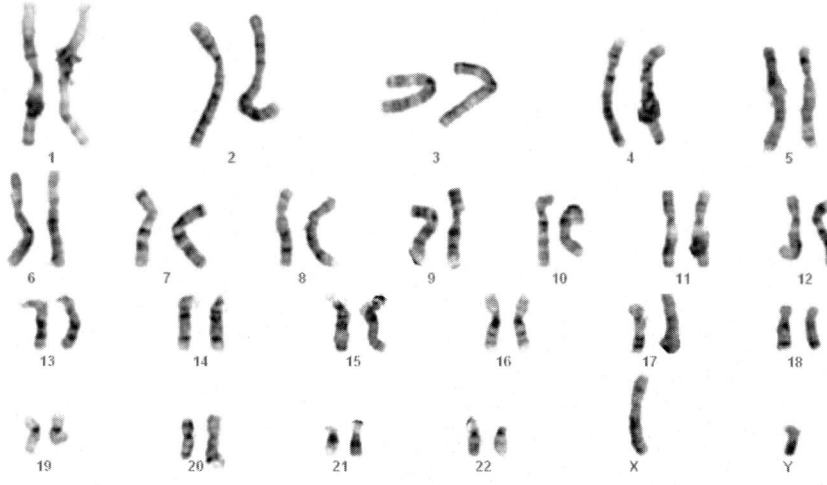

Figure 2. Human male karyotype. Normal male karyotype: 46,XY. Karyotype courtesy of the laboratory of Dr. Fern Tsien, Louisiana University Health Sciences Center Department of Genetics, used with permission.

Males can pass on either an X or a Y chromosome, which is why fathers are described as the sex-determining parent. The remaining chromosomes are autosomes, denoted by numbers 1 through 22. They are arranged into karyotypes by descending size, with 1 being the largest, and the sex chromosomes at the end. Chromosome 21 is the smallest chromosome. (Because of the difficulty visualizing chromosomes with early staining methods, chromosomes 21 and 22 were mistakenly put in reverse order. This assignment has remained.) A normal male karyotype is shown in Figure 2.

3. PATTERNS OF INHERITANCE

The four major patterns of inheritance are autosomal dominant, autosomal recessive, X-linked, and mitochondrial. These are each described in more detail in this section. *Autosomal* and *X-linked* both indicate the type of chromosome involved. X-linked genes are located on the X chromosome. Autosomal genes are located anywhere on chromosomes 1 to 22. Traits or disorders can be *dominant* or *recessive*. In Section 2.3, we learned that for any given gene (with the exception of mitochondrial genes), we inherit two copies: one from our mother and one from our father. These alternative gene copies are *alleles*. Alleles can interact in different ways. If one allele masks the other allele, it is a dominant allele. In contrast, a recessive allele is one that is capable of being masked by another allele. The combination of alleles inherited represents an individual's *genotype* while the expression of the genetic make-up represents an individual's *phenotype*. Alleles which differ from the norm may be deemed *mutations* or *polymorphisms*. Mutations typically describe allele variants which are disease-causing, while polymorphisms describe benign allele variants, though technically, the terms can be used interchangeably. Figures 3-7 show pedigrees of families with genetic deafness of different inheritance patterns. A pedigree is a diagrammatic representation of a family used by genetic counselors and clinical geneticists to record and evaluate genetic traits. In our examples we will use the trait of hearing loss.

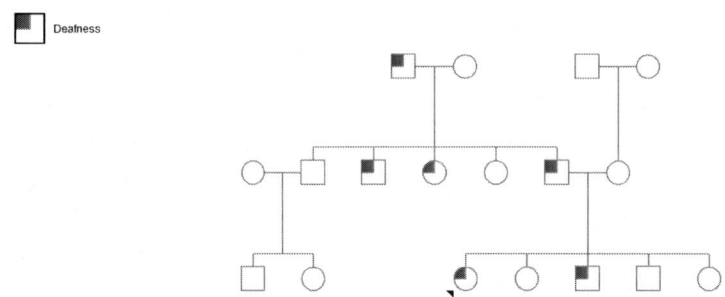

Figure 3. Pedigree of autosomal dominant deafness. Three generations of a family are shown in this pedigree. Males are represented by squares, females by circles; matings are denoted by a horizontal line, offspring by a vertical line. The proband (presenting patient) is indicated with an arrow. Family members affected with deafness are indicated with shading. For someone with autosomal dominant deafness, approximately half of their children would be expected to be deaf. Males and females are affected in roughly equal numbers.

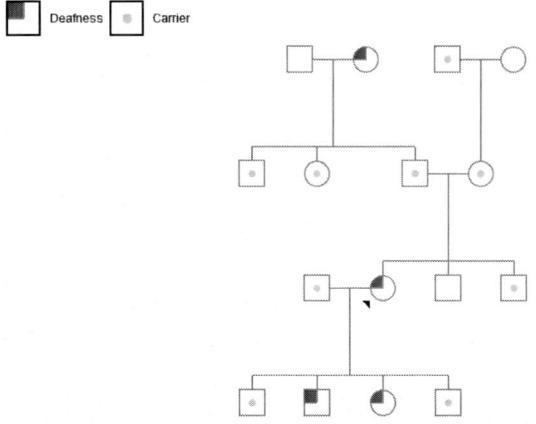

Figure 4. Pedigree of autosomal recessive deafness. Four generations of a family are shown in this pedigree. Males are represented by squares, females by circles; matings are denoted by a horizontal line, offspring by a vertical line. The proband (presenting patient) is indicated with an arrow. Family members affected with deafness are indicated with shading. Unaffected carriers are indicated with a dot. Deaf family members inherited two gene copies for deafness: one from each parent. For unaffected parents who are both carriers for autosomal recessive deafness in the same gene, approximately one-quarter of their children would be expected to be deaf. Males and females are affected in roughly equal numbers.

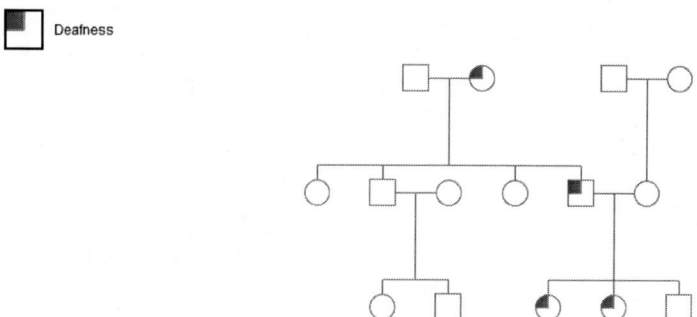

Figure 5. Pedigree of X-linked dominant deafness. Three generations of a family are shown in this pedigree. Males are represented by squares, females by circles; matings are denoted by a horizontal line, offspring by a vertical line. The proband (presenting patient) is indicated with an arrow. Family members affected with deafness are indicated with shading. Affected males will have all daughters affected and no sons affected. For affected females, half of their children will be affected (by probability) regardless of gender. X-linked inheritance will not display male-to-male transmission.

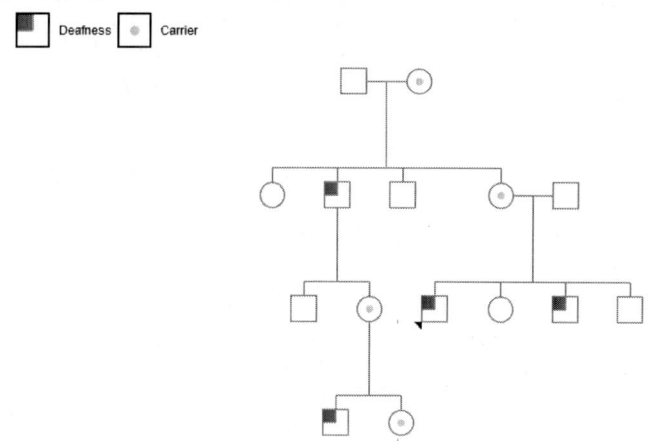

Figure 6. Pedigree of X-linked recessive deafness. Four generations of a family are shown in this pedigree. Males are represented by squares, females by circles; matings are denoted by a horizontal line, offspring by a vertical line. The proband (presenting patient) is indicated with an arrow. Family members affected with deafness are indicated with shading. Unaffected carriers are indicated with a dot. Those affected are disproportionately (sometimes exclusively) male. Carrier females may be affected (usually mildly) if X-inactivation is skewed toward the X chromosome with the normal allele. Affected males will pass the deafness gene to all of their daughters and none of their sons. Affected females will pass the gene on to half of their children (by probability), which is expected to result in all of their sons being affected and all of their daughters being carriers. X-linked inheritance will not display male-to-male transmission.

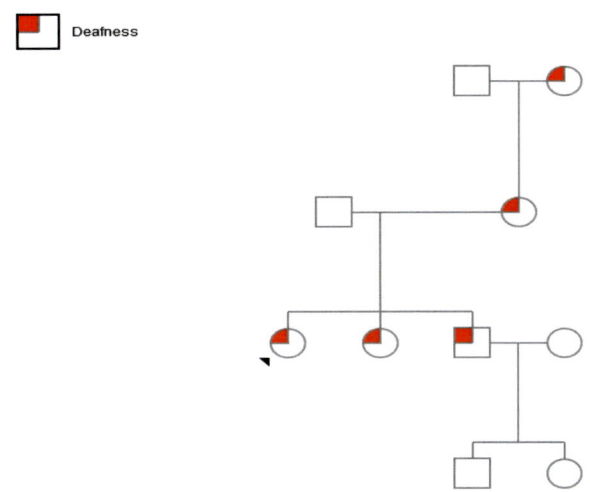

Figure 7. Pedigree of mitochondrial deafness. Four generations of a family are shown in this pedigree. Males are represented by squares, females by circles; matings are denoted by a horizontal line, offspring by a vertical line. The proband (presenting patient) is indicated with an arrow. Family members affected with deafness are indicated with shading. Affected females will pass the gene on to all of their children, while affected males will pass the gene on to none of their children. Males and females are affected in roughly equal numbers.

3.1. Autosomal Dominant

When a given trait or condition displays an autosomal dominant inheritance pattern, only one copy of a gene is necessary to cause the given trait. A person with autosomal dominant hearing loss will be expected to have received one copy of a hearing loss gene from one parent and a normal copy from the other parent. A parent with a mutation for autosomal dominant hearing loss will have a 50% chance of passing on the mutation to each child (Figure 8). Since the trait is dominant, we expect that each child receiving this allele will be affected with hearing loss. However, this is not always the case because some autosomal dominant traits exhibit reduced penetrance. If a trait is fully penetrant, all individuals who receive the allele will exhibit the trait.

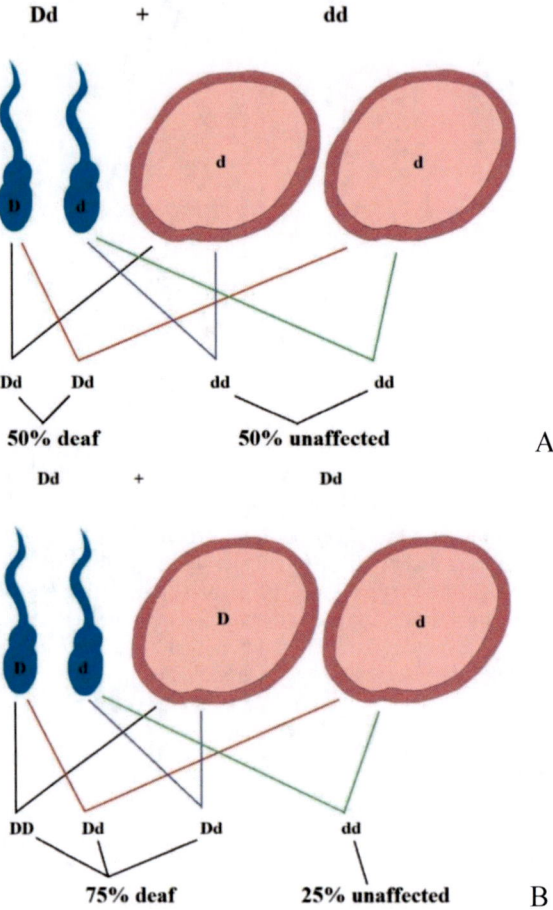

Figure 8. Autosomal dominant inheritance: risk to offspring. Autosomal dominant inheritance most commonly occurs when one parent is affected. In 8A, the father is affected with autosomal dominant deafness. We will use capital "D" and lowercase "d" to represent the dominant and recessive alleles for the gene in question, respectively. Since this gene is autosomal dominant, "D" is the deafness allele and "d" is the normal allele. The deaf father carries a "D" allele and a "d" allele, and therefore his sperm cells will be one of two varieties. Each of his children will inherit either a "D" allele or a "d" allele from him. There is a 50% chance of each of these possibilities for each child. The unaffected mother has two "d" alleles, and thus all of her children will inherit the "d" allele from her. Since the "D" allele is dominant and will result in deafness, 50% of the children born to this couple will be expected to exhibit deafness. In 8B, both parents have autosomal dominant deafness for the same gene. Both of them have one "D" allele and one "d" allele they can pass on to their children. When we evaluate each of the four combinations in which these alleles can come together, each child born to this union would have a 75% chance of being deaf (DD or Dd) and a 25% chance of being unaffected (dd).

If the trait has reduced penetrance, there will be individuals who carry the allele but do not possess the trait. It is not clear why this occurs, but it may be due to the influence of other genes. In a minority of cases of autosomal dominant hearing loss, the hearing loss arises due to a new mutation in the patient. When this occurs, neither parent will carry the mutation, and the odds of having another child with the same mutation are very low. This is why genetic testing of parents is necessary to estimate recurrence risks. While new mutations can occur in any type of disorder, they are seen far more frequently in autosomal dominant disorders because only one mutation is necessary.

3.2. Autosomal Recessive

A person with autosomal recessive hearing loss will have two copies of a mutation for the involved gene. Unlike dominant conditions, two copies are required for a recessive condition to appear. Those who carry one copy of a recessive gene are known as carriers because they do not show outward signs of the mutation they carry. The frequent mechanism of inheritance for an individual with autosomal recessive hearing loss is two unaffected parents who each carry a mutation for the causative gene. This is by far the most common scenario in genetic hearing loss, and explains in large part why more than 90% of children with permanent hearing loss are born to hearing parents [12]. Each child of parents who are carriers for mutations in the same gene will have a 25% chance of inheriting both copies, and therefore being affected. They will have a 50% chance of being an unaffected carrier (Figure 9). While new mutations can occur in recessive conditions, this is seen far less frequently because it would be unusual for two new mutations to occur in the same gene. Another slightly more probable mechanism has been observed in autosomal recessive disorders, whereby an individual receives one copy of a disease gene from one parent and experiences a new mutation in the same gene inherited from the other parent.

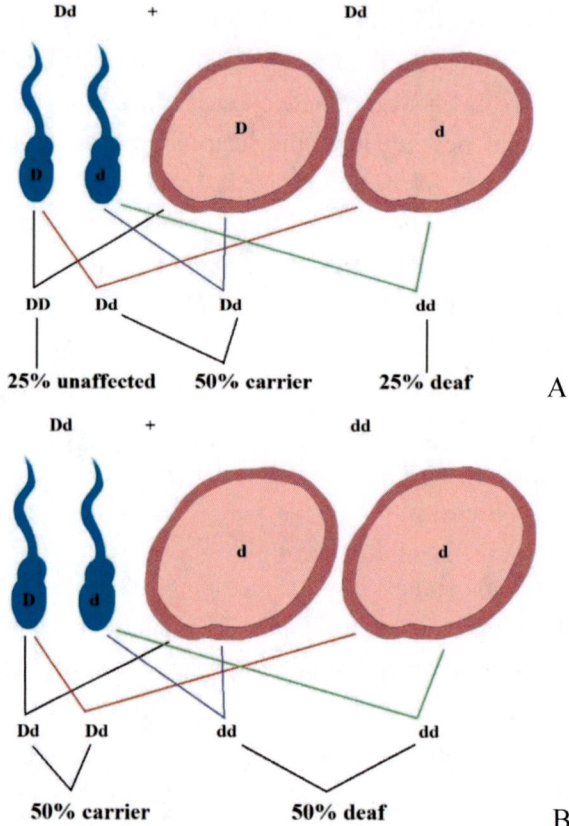

Figure 9. Autosomal recessive inheritance: risk to offspring. In autosomal recessive inheritance, the deafness gene is the lowercase "d". Deafness will only manifest if an individual carries both copies of the "d" deafness allele. Autosomal recessive inheritance most commonly occurs when two unaffected parents are carriers (9A). Both parents have the genotype Dd and can pass on either allele to each child. The four combinations possible from this union lead to a 25% chance of a deaf child (dd), a 50% chance of a child who is a carrier (Dd), and a 25% chance of an unaffected child (DD) from each conception. In 9B, the mother is affected with autosomal recessive deafness and the father is an unaffected carrier for the same gene. In this mating, each child has a 50% chance of being deaf (dd) and a 50% chance of being an unaffected carrier (Dd).

3.3. X-Linked

X-linked genes are inherited on the X chromosome, and are thus also known as sex-linked genes because they are inherited differently in males and females. Males are far more likely to exhibit an X-linked disorder, and they tend to be more severely affected than their female counterparts. Males are more vulnerable to X-linked disorders because they only possess one X chromosome. By having one X chromosome, males only have one copy of each gene located on the X-chromosome. Females have two X chromosomes, so a second allele could potentially mask a mutation on the other allele. For males, X-linked traits are maternally-inherited because males only inherit X chromosomes from their mothers. Likewise, a male with an X-linked disorder will pass this trait on to all of his daughters and none of his sons (Figure 10). X-linked genes can also be dominant or recessive, but some clinicians prefer not to use these descriptors because dominance and recessiveness are not as clear-cut with X-linked inheritance. When considering males, they will be affected with an X-linked disorder if they receive a gene with a mutation associated with a disorder. Since males will only have one copy of this gene, it is not particularly relevant to their condition whether or not it is dominant or recessive (though it may have relevance in regards to recurrence risks to offspring).

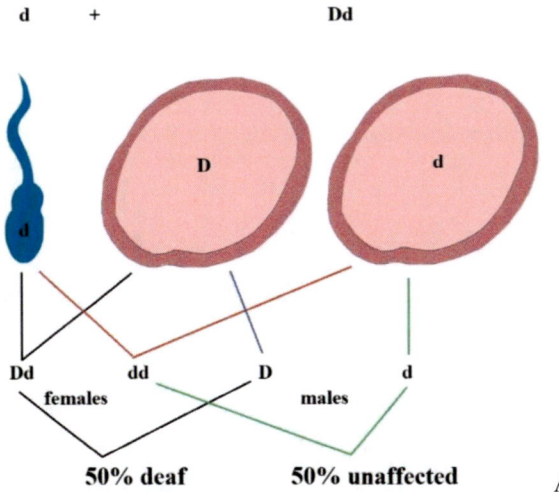

Figure 10. (Continued).

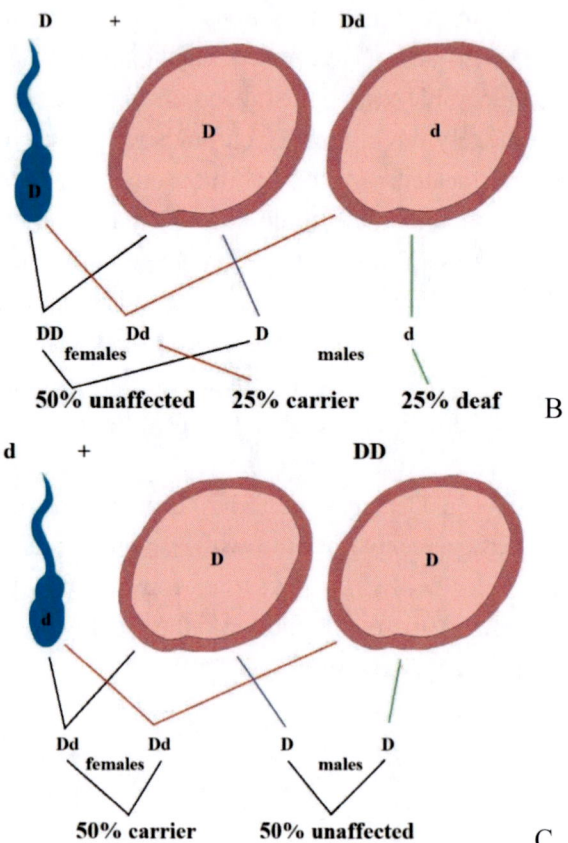

Figure 10. X-linked inheritance: risk to offspring. With X-linked inheritance, females have two X chromosomes, and therefore two alleles, while males have one X chromosome and one allele. 10A demonstrates X-linked dominant inheritance with an affected mother. The deafness allele is capital "D". The mother can pass on "D" or "d" to each of her children. The father can only pass on "d" to his daughters; he does not pass on an allele from the X chromosome to his sons because his sons will inherit a Y chromosome from him. Each child from this mating will have a 50% chance of being affected (Dd for daughters and D for sons) and a 50% chance of being unaffected (dd for daughters and d for sons). 10B illustrates X-linked recessive inheritance with a carrier mother (Dd) and an unaffected father (D). Since this is recessive inheritance, "d" is the deafness allele, which will only manifest in the absence of a "D". Sons can receive either "D" or "d" from their mother, and thus have a 50% chance of being deaf and a 50% chance of being unaffected. Since daughters can only receive a normal allele from their father, they will have a 50% chance of being a carrier (Dd) and a 50% chance of being unaffected (DD). Combining all offspring together for this mating, we expect 25% to be deaf, 25% to be carriers, and 50% to be unaffected. Finally in 10C, we have X-linked recessive inheritance with a deaf father (d) and an unaffected (noncarrier) mother (DD). In this mating all daughters will be carriers (Dd) and all sons will be unaffected (D).

Dominance and recessiveness have greater relevance with females, who have two X chromosomes. It would therefore be expected that a female would be affected with an X-linked dominant disorder if she carries one copy of the mutation, and would be affected with an X-linked recessive disorder only if she carries two copies of the mutation. However, there are cases of unaffected or mildly affected females with a mutation for an X-linked dominant disorder, as well as cases of affected females for an X-linked recessive disorder who carry only one copy of a mutation. This is due to a phenomenon known as skewed X-inactivation. During development, one of the X chromosomes in every cell of a female's body is inactivated. The X chromosome inactivated in each cell is largely random. As a result, females carrying one copy of an X-linked disease gene display wide variability depending on the proportions of inactivation for each X chromosome. It is because of skewed X-inactivation that an X-linked disorder that is dominant or recessive may not always appear to be inherited in a family as expected. It should also be noted that some X-linked disorders are actually more common in females. These tend to be X-linked dominant disorders with a severe clinical presentation. An example is Rett syndrome, characterized by severe developmental delay and autistic features. Rett syndrome is inherited on the X chromosome, but it is observed almost exclusively in females because it is lethal to males *in utero*. A similar outcome occurs in many autosomal dominant disorders when two mutation copies are inherited.

3.4. Mitochondrial

Mitochondria are cellular organelles primarily responsible for energy production, hence their nickname "powerhouse of the cell." The mitochondria are located outside the nucleus, where the chromosomes are located (Figure 11). Mitochondria have their own genome of only 37 genes located on one circular chromosome whose structure and function are reminiscent of a bacterial chromosome. Mitochondria are found in many cells throughout the body, including egg cells, but they are not found in mature sperm cells. Because they are not in sperm cells, mitochondrial genes are exclusively inherited maternally. A mother with a mutation in a mitochondrial gene will pass on the mutation to all of her children, while a man with a mitochondrial mutation will not pass it on to any of his children (Figure 12). The primitive mitochondrial genome does not have the sophisticated DNA repair mechanisms observed in the nuclear genome, and thus, is highly prone to mutations.

4. SYNDROMIC HEARING LOSS

A syndrome is a disease, disorder, or condition that is associated with a particular set of signs, symptoms, or characteristics. Though many syndromes have a genetic etiology, this is not always the case.

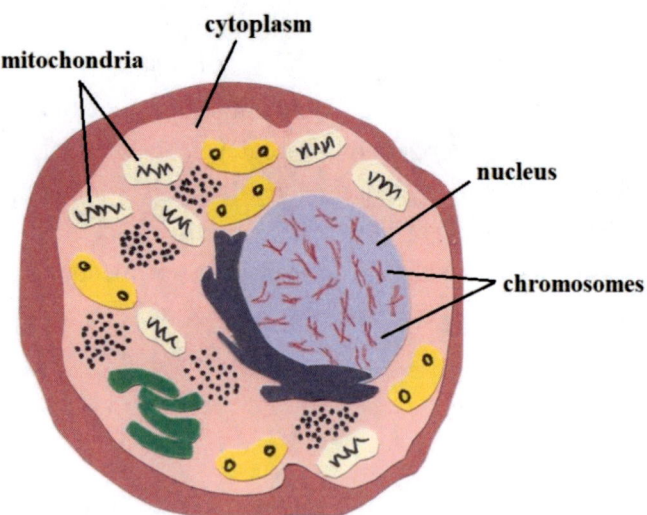

Figure 11. Human Cell. This figure illustrates the position of the nuclear and mitochondrial genomes in the human cell. The nucleus contains 46 chromosomes (23 chromosomes in gametes), which hold nearly all of the approximately 20,000 human genes. Mitochondria are organelles located in the cytoplasm, outside of the nucleus. Mitochondria have their own genome consisting of 37 genes. The inheritance of these genes does not follow the same inheritance pattern as nuclear genes. Rather, mitochondrial genes are inherited exclusively from the mother, as they are found in egg cells but not in sperm cells.

Genetics of Hearing Loss

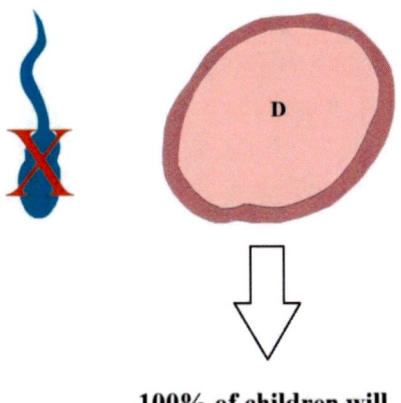

100% of children will receive mother's D allele

Figure 12. Mitochondrial inheritance: risk to offspring. Since mature sperm cells do not contain mitochondria, a father's genotype for a mitochondrial gene has no effect on his offspring. A mother who is affected with a mitochondrial gene will pass this on to all of her children. (Though not discussed in this chapter, mitochondrial inheritance is sometimes more complex than this. An individual can carry mitochondria which are all of the same genotype, known as *homoplasmy*, or mitochondria with different genotypes, known as *heteroplasmy*. Homoplasmy is demonstrated here.)

Syndromic hearing loss is a syndrome which typically includes hearing loss as one of its clinical features. While many syndromes are characterized by distinct facial or physical features, bear in mind that clinical features are not always readily visible. Below is a brief overview of selected syndromes with hearing loss as a clinical feature in many patients.

4.1. Syndromes with Autosomal Dominant Inheritance

4.1.1. Stickler Syndrome

Stickler syndrome has an incidence of 1 in 7,500 to 9,000. It is associated with visual problems, which may include severe nearsightedness, glaucoma, cataracts, and retinal detachment. There is a characteristic flattened facial appearance, which often includes a large tongue, small lower jaw, and cleft palate. Joints are very flexible.

Conductive, sensorineural, or mixed hearing loss may be seen, as the middle ear and inner ear can be affected [13, 14].

Stickler syndrome is inherited in an autosomal dominant fashion, though a small number of cases are inherited in an autosomal recessive fashion or are due to new mutations. It is caused by mutations in various genes which code for collagen proteins: *COL2A1*, *COL9A1*, *COL11A1*, and *COL11A2* [14]. The abnormal collagen causes the bones of the face to not form properly and leads to hyperflexibility in the joints. Breathing and feeding difficulties result from the combination of a large tongue and small lower jaw. Hearing loss is usually present at birth and gets worse over time [13, 14].

4.1.2. CHARGE Syndrome

CHARGE syndrome is a serious medical disorder characterized by a number of physical and developmental problems and distinct facial features. It has an incidence of 1 in 10,000. It was originally named for what was believed to be its major features: *C*oloboma, *H*eart defects, *A*tresia of choanae, *R*etardation of growth and development, *G*enital and/or urinary abnormalities, and *E*ar abnormalities and deafness. Many patients are born with life-threatening birth defects, such as heart defects and breathing problems. Intelligence is variable but most patients have severe intellectual disability. Choanal atresia or stenosis (narrow or blocked passages from the back of the nose to the throat) cause breathing problems. Cranial nerve abnormalities may be present, especially of nerves I, VII, and IX/X, leading to absent or decreased sense of smell, facial palsy, and swallowing difficulties, respectively. Coloboma of the eye (cleft of the iris, retina, choroids, macula, or disc) may be associated with vision loss. Cleft lip and/or palate, kidney problems, and tracheo-esophageal fistula may be present [15, 16].

The outer, middle, and inner ear can all be affected, and thus hearing loss may be conductive, sensorineural, or mixed. Severity of hearing loss ranges from mild to profound and may be progressive. Outer ear abnormalities reported include a short, wide pinna with little or no lobe, triangular concha, decreased cartilage leading to a floppy ear, and a missing piece of helix, giving the appearance that a piece of the helix has been snipped. Malformed ossicles have been reported in the middle ear, as well as chronic, recurrent otitis media with effusion. Mondini defects and small or absent semicircular canals may occur in the inner ear [15, 16].

Characteristic facies are a square face with a broad prominent forehead, arched eyebrows, ptosis, flat midface, small mouth, facial asymmetry, and prominent nasal bridge with square root. A common physical feature is a palmar crease in the shape of a hockey stick [15, 16].

CHARGE syndrome is caused by a mutation in the *CHD7* gene. *CHD7* helps regulate gene expression during development. A mutation in this gene causes disrupted development, resulting in many physical abnormalities. Only about 2/3 of patients test positive for a *CHD7* mutation, so there may be other causative genes that have not been identified. Diagnosis is most frequently made clinically. Inheritance pattern is autosomal dominant, but almost all cases are due to new mutations. Recurrence risks are therefore very low for parents with an affected child [17-20].

4.1.3. Cornelia de Lange Syndrome

The exact incidence of Cornelia de Lange syndrome is unknown, but it is estimated at 1 in 10,000 to 30,000. Clinical presentation is variable from one patient to the next, but there are many physical signs associated with Cornelia de Lange syndrome, including: severe to profound intellectual disability and growth retardation, microcephaly, hirsutism, confluent eyebrows, small nose with anteverted nares, downturned upper lip, micrognathia, long curly eyelashes, cleft palate, cardiac defects, and severely malformed upper limbs, possibly with missing fingers or toes and webbed toes. Auditory system defects may include low-set auricles and small external auditory canals. Hearing loss is variable and may be conductive, sensorineural, or mixed [21, 22].

Cornelia de Lange syndrome has been reported to be caused by mutations in five different genes: *NIPBL*, *SMC1A*, *HDAC8*, *RAD21*, and *SMC3* [23-26]. Mutations in *NIPBL* are responsible for more than half of cases. These genes code for proteins important for prenatal growth development. The cause is unknown in about 30% of cases, suggesting there are more genes yet to be identified. Inheritance pattern is typically autosomal dominant, though approximately 5% of cases are X-linked dominant. Most cases are due to new mutations, and thus occur in patients with no family history [23-26].

4.1.4. Neurofibromatosis Type 2

Neurofibromatosis type 2 (NF2) is a disorder featuring growth of benign tumors in the nervous system, primarily in the brain. In many patients this includes growths on one or both vestibulocochlear nerves. These vestibular schwannomas/acoustic neuromas lead to the same sequelae as patients without NF2: neural hearing loss, tinnitus, and vertigo. A notable difference is that a patient with NF2 is likely to be affected bilaterally, though not necessarily at the same time. In those affected bilaterally, loss of VIIIth nerve function is common [27, 28]. If loss of VIIIth nerve function is bilateral, the patient is not a cochlear implant candidate but may pursue an auditory brainstem implant. However, auditory brainstem implant outcomes have been reported to be poorer for NF2 patients compared with non-NF2 patients [29]. Other NF2 tumors may cause vision changes, peripheral numbness or weakness, or fluid in the brain. The incidence of NF2 is estimated at 1 in 33,000. Signs often show up in childhood, though they can develop at any age [27, 28].

NF2 is caused by mutations in the *NF2* gene, which codes for a protein important for insulating neurons [30]. NF2 is an autosomal dominant disorder, but it is inherited from an affected parent in only half of cases. The remainder are due to new mutations. NF2 should not be confused with the more common neurofibromatosis type 1 (NF1, incidence of 1 in 4,000), which is not typically associated with hearing loss. Physical signs of NF1 include café-au-lait spots (areas of darker pigmentation on the skin), Lisch nodules (growths on the iris of the eyes), axillary and inguinal freckling, subcutaneous neurofibromas, and optic gliomas, which may lead to vision loss [27, 28].

4.1.5. Branchio-oto-Renal Syndrome

Branchio-oto-renal syndrome affects the neck (branchio), the ears (oto), and the kidneys (renal). Estimated prevalence of this syndrome is 1 in 40,000. This syndrome arises from a disruption in the development of tissues in the neck. Primary physical signs include branchial cleft cysts, fistulae between the skin of the neck and the throat, preauricular pits or tags, malformed or misshapen pinnae, middle or inner ear structural defects, and abnormal kidney structure and function [31, 32]. Surgery may be warranted to treat cysts or fistulae of the neck. Dialysis may be needed to treat kidney disease. Hearing loss can vary in severity, and may be conductive, sensorineural, or mixed. Approximately 2% of the profoundly deaf are thought to have branchio-oto-renal syndrome [33].

Mutations in three different genes have been reported to cause branchio-oto-renal syndrome: *EYA1*, *SIX1*, and *SIX5*, with *EYA1* being responsible for about 40% of cases [34-36]. The resultant proteins from these genes are involved in embryonic development. Branchio-oto-renal syndrome is inherited in an autosomal dominant fashion. About 10% of cases are due to new mutations [37].

4.1.6. Waardenburg Syndrome

Waardenburg syndrome consists of sensorineural hearing loss along with specific physical features, including a white forelock; pale blue eyes, different-colored eyes (complete heterochromia), or two different colors in the same eye (partial heterochromia); widely-spaced eyes (hypertelorism); lateral displacement of medial canthi; prominent broad nasal root; and hypertrichosis of the medial part of the eyebrows [38, 39]. Its prevalence is estimated at 1 in 42,000 [39]. Hearing loss severity can range from mild to profound, and is usually bilateral, though unilateral cases have been reported [40]. Some individuals will show physical features but have normal hearing. About 2% of cases of profound congenital hearing loss are attributable to Waardenburg syndrome [38].

There are four distinct types of Waardenburg, with types I and II being the most common. Physical features vary between types but also between individuals of the same type. For example, hypertelorism is commonly seen in type I and not in type II, while hearing loss is more common in type II than in type I [41]. Waardenburg syndrome exhibits reduced penetrance, meaning individuals who carry a mutation for Waardenburg syndrome do not always manifest the disorder. These individuals can, however, pass it on to their children where it may be fully penetrant in the offspring. This syndrome also demonstrates variable expressivity, meaning that individuals with the same mutation may have different clinical presentations. This can even occur in members of the same family. Inheritance pattern is typically autosomal dominant, but a small number of cases are due to autosomal recessive inheritance or new mutations. Several genes have been implicated in Waardenburg syndrome, many of which are involved in melanocyte development [42]. The reader is referred to OMIM (Online Mendelian Inheritance in Man) at https://www.omim.org/ for a current review [43].

4.1.7. Treacher Collins Syndrome

Treacher Collins syndrome has an incidence of 1 in 50,000 live births. This condition arises from abnormal development of facial bones and tissues. Characteristic facial features include down-slanting palpebral fissures, notched lower eyelids, micrognathia, underdevelopment or absence of cheekbones and eye socket floor, and cleft palate. About half of individuals with Treacher Collins syndrome have conductive hearing loss due to atresia, microtia, and/or malformed ossicles [44, 45].

Most cases of Treacher Collins syndrome display autosomal dominant inheritance, but less than 2% show autosomal recessive inheritance. Approximately 60% of autosomal dominant cases are due to new mutations. More than 80% of cases are due to the *TCOF1* gene, with a small minority due to *POLR1C* and *POLR1D* [46, 47]. These genes play roles in the development of facial bones and tissues. Variable expressivity is seen in Treacher Collins syndrome ranging from unnoticeable to severe facial malformation [48]. Because of this, it should not be assumed that a patient's Treacher Collins syndrome is due to a new mutation when neither of the parents exhibit signs of the condition. Patients and their parents should receive genetics evaluations if the families desire accurate estimates of recurrence risks.

4.1.8. Crouzon Syndrome

Crouzon syndrome is the most common craniosynostosis disorder, with an incidence of 1 in 60,000 live births. Facial features include midface hypoplasia, shallow orbits with protruding eyes, strabismus, beaked nose, underdeveloped upper jaw, and large forehead. Dental problems and cleft lip and palate are also common. Conductive hearing loss occurs due to deformed or narrow external ear canals, narrowed internal auditory canals, chronic otitis media with effusion, and poor Eustachian tube function [49, 50].

Crouzon syndrome is caused by mutations in the *FGFR2* gene. This gene has many functions, including signaling cellular differentiation during embryonic development [50]. Mutations lead to premature fusion of sutures in the skull. Inheritance for Crouzon syndrome is autosomal dominant, though approximately 25% of cases are due to new mutations [51].

4.1.9. Apert Syndrome

Apert syndrome is a craniosynostosis disorder with many similarities to Crouzon syndrome. Reported incidence and prevalence data vary, but Apert syndrome affects approximately 1 in 70,000 live births with a prevalence of about 1 in 100,000. Common physical features are frontal bossing, midface hypoplasia, protruding eyes, strabismus, low-set ears, syndactyly, hyperhidrosis, oily skin with severe acne, patches of missing hair in the eyebrows, and cleft lip and palate. Shallow eye sockets can cause vision problems. Cognitive abilities range from normal to mild to moderate intellectual disability. Conductive hearing loss and recurrent otitis media are common [49, 52].

Like Crouzon syndrome, Apert syndrome is caused by mutations in the *FGFR2* gene and has an autosomal dominant inheritance pattern. Unlike Crouzon syndrome, virtually all cases of Apert syndrome are due to new mutations [49, 52].

4.2. Syndromes with Autosomal Recessive Inheritance

4.2.1. Pendred Syndrome

Pendred syndrome is a disorder associated with sensorineural hearing loss and thyroid goiter. Exact incidence is unknown but it is estimated to affect 1 in 13,000 to 15,000 people. Thyroid goiter is most likely to appear between late childhood and early adulthood, and it usually does not affect thyroid function. Severe to profound sensorineural hearing loss is typically congenital and may be progressive or fluctuating. Enlarged vestibular aqueduct is typically present, which may cause balance disturbances [53-55]. About half of individuals with Pendred syndrome have a Mondini malformation [55].

Pendred syndrome is caused by mutations in the *SLC26A4* gene, which codes for pendrin, a protein that transports anions in and out of cells. While its role is not fully understood, it is known to be important for normal functioning of the thyroid and inner ear [56]. Inheritance of Pendred syndrome is autosomal recessive. Mutations in *SLC26A4* are also responsible for some cases of nonsyndromic hearing loss. Altogether this gene is thought to account for 5 to 10% of hereditary deafness [57, 58].

4.2.2. Usher Syndrome

Usher syndrome is a condition of combined hearing loss and vision loss, sometimes accompanied by vestibular dysfunction. Its prevalence worldwide is estimated at 4 per 100,000, but it is reported to be much more common in certain populations, particularly in Ashkenazi Jewish and Louisiana Acadian populations [59, 60]. Though rare, Usher syndrome is responsible for about half of all concurrent deafness and blindness in adults [61, 62]. There are three types of Usher syndrome, with type I being the most severe. Vision loss first presents as night blindness and later progresses to retinitis pigmentosa [59].

The typical course for type I Usher syndrome is congenital bilateral profound sensorineural deafness, with progressive vision loss beginning around 10 years of age [59]. The vision deteriorates to blindness by early adulthood. There is also an absence of vestibular function, which frequently goes unnoticed. Mothers of children with Usher syndrome commonly report they were late to begin walking, often 18 months to 2 years of age. As the child grows and develops, the central nervous system adapts to this lack of vestibular function. A typical presentation of type II Usher syndrome is congenital moderate to severe sensorineural hearing loss, and vision loss beginning in adolescence [63]. Progression to blindness commonly occurs in the 30s. Vestibular function remains intact. Type III is the mildest form of Usher syndrome. It accounts for only 2-4% of cases worldwide, but up to 40% of cases in the Finnish population [63]. Hearing loss is progressive and typically less severe. Onset of both hearing loss and retinitis pigmentosa is variable. Vestibular function among patients is also variable, with everything from normal to absent vestibular function reported. A summary of Usher syndrome clinical presentations by type is shown in Table 1.

Table 1. Usher syndrome clinical presentations by type

	Type I	Type II	Type III
Hearing Loss	Profound	Severe	Progressive
Vestibular function	Absent	Normal	Variable
Onset of blindness (decade)	First	Second	Variable

Usher syndrome is an autosomal recessive disorder. It is thought to be more common in certain populations, such as the Louisiana Acadians, due to the founder effect, illustrated in Figure 13 [60]. A founder effect results when a small group of individuals become "founders" of a new population. This new founder population becomes isolated, either geographically or culturally, from other populations for several generations. The ultimate effect is that they become genetically isolated. Since the original founders were from a very small group, they may not be genetically diverse. After many generations certain traits or disorders may be amplified. In the case of the Louisiana Acadians, their roots can be traced back to French descendants of Canadian Nova Scotia Acadians. A few hundred of these descendants migrated to southern Louisiana in the 1700s. At this writing there are 11 genes associated with Usher syndrome and 3 genetic loci [63].

A locus is a fixed position on a chromosome, in this case where a gene is located. A locus (plural loci) may be described in association with a certain trait or condition prior to the identification of the responsible gene. Hence, there will likely be more genes recognized as causative for Usher syndrome. Genes responsible for Usher syndrome code for proteins of different classes and families. For more information on the functions of these proteins, the reader is referred to Yan and Liu, 2010 [63]. The genes involved in Usher syndrome are listed in Table 2.

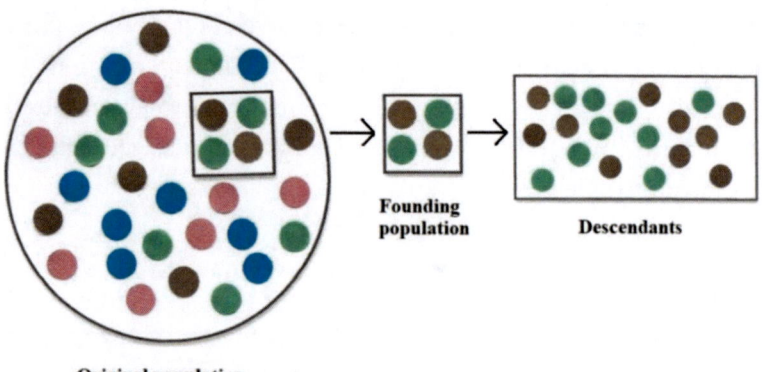

Figure 13. Founder effect. The founder effect is observed when a population is derived from a founding population which consisted of relatively few members. This figure illustrates the concept of the founder effect. A few members of the original larger population broke off and formed a new colony. Due to the small starting population size, the colony has reduced genetic variation and a non-random sample of the genes from the original population. After many generations of geographic and cultural isolation, gene variants which were once rare have propagated and become relatively common. As a result, some diseases are found more frequently in these groups than in other populations, or they have distinct clinical or genetic features due to unique mutations.

Table 2. Genes involved in Usher syndrome

Type I	Type II	Type III
MYO7A	USH2A	USH3A
USH1C	ADGRV1	HARS
CDH23	WHRN	
PCD15		
SANS		
CIB2		

4.2.3. Jervell and Lange-Nielsen Syndrome

Jervell and Lange-Nielsen syndrome affects 1.6 to 6 per 1,000,000 people. Though rare, it has been suggested that up to 3 out of 1,000 people born deaf have Jervell and Lange-Nielsen syndrome [64]. It is characterized by congenital bilateral profound sensorineural hearing loss and cardiac defects. Since the cardiac issues are not present at birth, a proper diagnosis is often late or missed altogether. The first physical signs of cardiac problems are irregular heartbeats in early childhood, which may lead to episodes of fainting, or syncope. Long QT syndrome, a serious condition causing heart muscle to take longer than usual to recharge between beats, may be present [65]. There is a risk of cardiac arrest and sudden death in patients with this syndrome. Treatment may involve beta-adrenergic blockers for long QT syndrome and implantable cardioverter defibrillators (ICDs) for patients with a history of cardiac arrest [66].

Jervell and Lange-Nielsen syndrome is caused by mutations in either the *KCNQ1* or *KCNE1* genes. *KCNQ1* is responsible for 90% of cases while *KCNE1* is responsible for 10% of cases [66]. These genes code for potassium ion channels. Mutations in one of these genes lead to faulty potassium ion channels, which disrupts the usual flow of ions through the inner ear and cardiac muscle. The heart and inner ear are the areas of the body with the greatest utilization of potassium ions. Therefore, these areas are most affected by the faulty channels [66]. Jervell and Lange-Nielsen syndrome is an autosomal recessive disorder.

4.3. Syndrome with X-Linked Inheritance: Alport Syndrome

Alport syndrome is characterized by hearing loss, kidney disease, and eye abnormalities, which may include a decrease in vision in a minority of patients [67]. It has a reported incidence of 1 in 50,000 [68]. Hearing loss varies from mild to severe sensorineural hearing loss, often sloping, and may be progressive. Typical age of onset for hearing loss is late childhood to early adolescence. More than half of patients with Alport syndrome have hearing loss, with males much more likely than females to exhibit this clinical feature. Kidney disease is preceded by blood in the urine (hematuria). As kidney disease progresses, proteinuria and hypertension develop. Many patients develop end-stage renal disease and require dialysis and kidney transplantation. Males are almost always more severely affected than females. Eye abnormalities may include anterior lenticonus (an abnormally-shaped lens), cataracts, corneal erosions, and retinal thinning [69].

Alport syndrome is caused by mutations in *COL4A3*, *COL4A4*, and *COL4A5*, genes coding for type IV collagen [70, 71]. This type of collagen is an important structural component in the glomeruli of the kidneys. Approximately 80 to 85% of cases are inherited in an X-linked dominant fashion, explaining why males are affected more frequently and more severely than females. About 15% of cases display an autosomal recessive inheritance pattern and 1% show an autosomal dominant pattern [72].

4.4. Syndromes with Mitochondrial Inheritance: MELAS and MERRF

MELAS and MERRF are two syndromes caused by mitochondrial mutations. The exact incidences of these syndromes are unknown, but they are both very rare. As with all mitochondrial disorders, they are inherited maternally, though they can be due to new mutations. MELAS and MERRF both affect many systems of the body, especially the muscles, brain, and nervous system, cell types rich in mitochondria [73, 74]. Severity is variable, sometimes even amongst affected family members. Sensorineural hearing loss can appear in both syndromes. They are named after their most prominent features: *MELAS* (*M*itochondrial *e*ncephalomyopathy, *L*actic *a*cidosis, and *S*troke-like episodes); *MERRF* (*M*yoclonic *e*pilepsy with *R*agged *r*ed *f*ibers). Muscle pain/weakness/twitches and seizures are common features [73, 74].

4.5. Down Syndrome: The Most Common Genetic Syndrome

Down syndrome occurs in 1 out of every 700 live births, making it the most common genetic syndrome [75]. Down syndrome differs from the other genetic syndromes discussed in this chapter in that it is a cytogenetic, or chromosomal disorder. Also known as trisomy 21, Down syndrome is caused by an extra chromosome 21. An individual with Down syndrome will therefore have a chromosome complement of 47 in every cell, as opposed to the typical 46 chromosomes. This is essentially a duplication of every gene on chromosome 21. (A minority of cases display mosaicism, in which some cells have 47 chromosomes and some cells have 46 chromosomes. These patients tend to be affected more mildly.) Chromosome 21 has over 700 genes, 200 to 300 of which code for proteins [76]. Down syndrome is one of the few trisomies that is compatible with life, owing to the fact that there are fewer genes on chromosome 21 than any other autosome. (The Y chromosome, a sex chromosome, contains about 200 fewer genes.)

Down syndrome consists of intellectual disability, characteristic facial and physical features, and heart defects in about half of patients. Physical features include hypotonia, flat facial profile, epicanthal folds, up-slanting palpebral fissures, small low-set ears with folded helix, shortened limbs, and transpalmar crease [77]. Gastrointestinal problems associated with intestinal or esophageal blockages may occur. There is an increased risk of developing heart disease and leukemia. Hearing loss is common, especially conductive hearing loss owing to small ear canals and short Eustachian tubes. These attributes frequently lead to cerumen blockage and chronic otitis media with effusion, respectively. Sensorineural hearing loss is also not uncommon in individuals with Down syndrome, with permanent hearing loss being reported in 25% of patients [78].

Down syndrome occurs during a nondisjunction event during cell division, whereby the homologous pair of chromosome 21s do not segregate appropriately into each daughter cell. This nondisjunction can occur via three different mechanisms: during meiosis of the egg cell, during meiosis of the sperm cell, or during postzygotic mitosis. Nondisjunction during meiosis of the egg cell is the most common mechanism, and is illustrated in Figure 14. It is unknown why nondisjunction occurs, but it happens much more frequently in egg cells as a woman ages. Advanced maternal age is therefore a major risk factor for Down syndrome. It can be diagnosed prenatally through cytogenetic testing via maternal blood sample (cell-free fetal DNA), amniocentesis, or chorionic villus sampling (CVS).

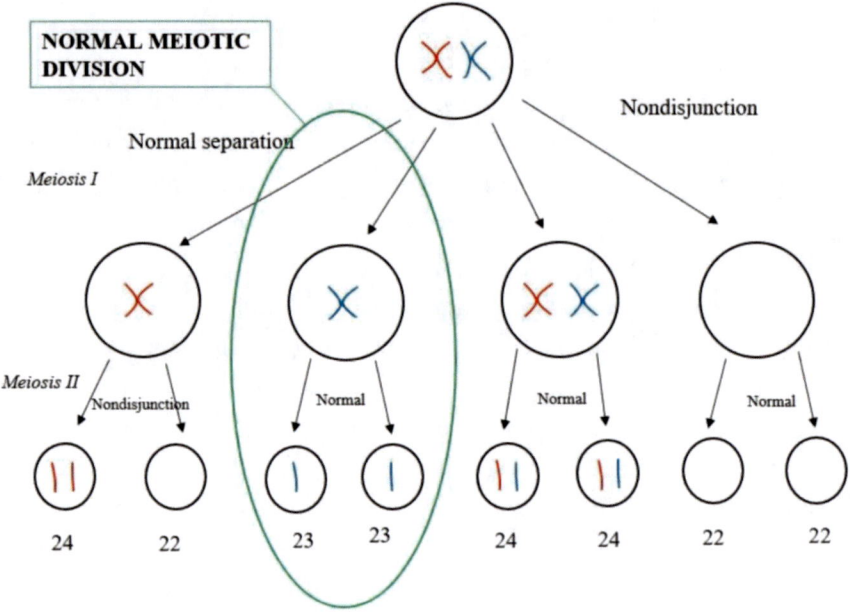

Figure 14. Chromosome nondisjunction during meiosis. Meiosis is cell division in gametes (egg and sperm cells). It consists of two cell divisions, vs. one cell division in mitosis (somatic cells). For simplicity, this figure shows one chromosome pair. (Human cells contain 23 chromosome pairs.) In meiosis I, the chromosome pair segregates into two separate cells. In meiosis II, the chromosome splits at the centromere, halving the genetic material. The process of meiosis II is similar to mitosis. The cells circled in green resulted from correct cell divisions. The remaining cells experienced a nondisjunction event in either meiosis I or meiosis II. Nondisjunction produces cells with too much or too little genetic material, which are almost always incompatible with life. However, excess genetic material can be compatible with life if the chromosome is very small, such as chromosome 21. An extra chromosome 21 is known as trisomy 21, or Down syndrome.

5. NONSYNDROMIC HEARING LOSS

Nonsyndromic hearing loss refers to hearing loss occurring in isolation, in the absence of other clinical features. In this context, we are referring to nonsyndromic hearing losses with genetic etiologies. However, the term "nonsyndromic hearing loss" may be used in cases of isolated hearing loss due to other etiologies or when the etiology is unknown. Bear in mind that many cases of nonsyndromic hearing loss of unknown etiology will in fact have a genetic etiology or a genetic contributor.

Approximately 70% of genetic hearing loss cases are nonsyndromic [79]. Of these genetic nonsyndromic cases, 75 to 80% show an autosomal recessive inheritance pattern, 20% show an autosomal dominant inheritance pattern, and 1 to 2% show an X-linked or mitochondrial inheritance pattern [79]. More than 100 genes have been identified as causative for nonsyndromic hearing loss. For the most up-to-date data, visit the Hereditary Hearing Loss Homepage [9].

5.1. Nonsyndromic Hearing Loss: Autosomal Recessive Inheritance

5.1.1. Connexin 26 Hearing Loss Is Caused by the GJB2 Gene

The most common cause of all forms of genetic nonsyndromic hearing loss is the *GJB2* gene, commonly known as connexin 26 [80]. You may also see it referred to as *DFNB1*, its locus name. Connexins are proteins that play supporting roles in the cochlea, and are thought to be important for the recycling of potassium ions in the cochlea [81]. Mutations in the *GJB2* gene are responsible for about half of all cases of autosomal recessive nonsyndromic hearing loss [80]. More than 100 mutations have been reported in this gene [82]. By far, the most common mutation is the 35delG mutation, accounting for about 70% of cases [83]. The 35delG mutation is found in populations all over the world, but it is most common in Caucasian populations, particularly those of northern European or Mediterranean descent [79, 84]. Likewise, this population has the highest carrier rate for the 35delG mutation. The carrier rate refers to the proportion of individuals in a given population who are carriers for a genetic trait or disorder. It generally is used to describe autosomal recessive conditions because carriers of an autosomal recessive condition will not be affected. As previously discussed in section 3.2, a carrier of an autosomal recessive disorder will not exhibit the disorder themselves because they only have one copy of the mutation. Their other gene copy, or allele, is normal, and thus protein function from this gene copy is normal. When a carrier passes on genes to their offspring, each child may get the normal copy or the affected copy, the 35delG mutation in this case. In populations where the carrier rate is high, there is a greater likelihood that two individuals who are carriers for the same disorder will mate. For the 35delG mutation, carrier rates are 2 to 3% for Caucasians, 4 to 5% for Ashkenazi Jewish, and 1% for Japanese [79, 84].

Connexin 26 hearing loss shows a great deal of clinical variability, likely a reflection of the many different mutations and populations in which it is found [80, 85]. As in most forms of autosomal recessive hearing loss, the hearing loss in connexin 26 tends to have an early onset. Hearing loss is usually present in early childhood and may be congenital. In many cases, the hearing loss remains stable, but some cases show a progressive worsening of hearing loss. The type of hearing loss is sensorineural, but the degree is variable. Individuals with connexin 26 can have anywhere from mild to profound hearing loss [85]. The degree of hearing loss can even vary between members of the same family. Both ears are usually affected to the same degree. Though far less common, autosomal dominant mutations in connexin 26 also exist.

5.1.2. Other Genes

There are too many genes associated with hearing loss to discuss here. What follows is a brief description of the next seven most common causative genes in autosomal recessive hearing loss. The reader is encouraged to further investigate any genes of interest on OMIM [43]. An exhaustive list can be accessed on the Hereditary Hearing Loss Homepage [9].

5.1.2.1. *SLC26A4*

SLC26A4 codes for pendrin. This is the same gene that causes Pendred syndrome, discussed in section 4.2.1, and thus, hearing loss configuration shows similarities to Pendred syndrome. Different mutations in this gene cause nonsyndromic hearing loss. Onset of hearing loss is prelingual, frequently congenital. Typical audiometric configuration is moderate to profound sensorineural hearing loss, affecting anywhere from high frequencies to all frequencies. Hearing loss may be fluctuating or progressive. As observed in occurrences of Pendred syndrome, most patients have an enlarged vestibular aqueduct. Mondini defects may be present in some patients [57, 58].

5.1.2.2. *MYO15A*

MYO15A codes for myosin 15A, one of the myosins, a group of motor proteins of many functions, some of which are important for the structure of stereocilia. Onset of hearing loss is prelingual, usually congenital. Typical audiometric configuration is severe to profound sensorineural hearing loss with all frequencies affected [86-88].

5.1.2.3. *OTOF*

The *OTOF* gene codes for otoferlin, a protein thought to be involved in vesicle membrane fusion. Onset of hearing loss is prelingual. This is the most common genetic cause of auditory neuropathy [89].

5.1.2.4. *CDH23*

CDH23, also known as cadherin 23, is another protein expressed in the stereocilia of hair cells [90, 91]. Onset of hearing loss is prelingual, and configuration is severe to profound sensorineural hearing loss. All frequencies are typically affected, but hearing loss may be seen in the high frequencies first [92]. Mutations in the CDH23 gene are also associated with Usher syndrome type 1D [90].

5.1.2.5. *TMC1*

The *TMC1* gene codes for transmembrane channel-like protein 1. The exact function of this gene is unknown, but it is required for normal function of cochlear hair cells. Autosomal recessive and autosomal dominant mutations have been reported. Hearing loss is usually congenital profound sensorineural with an autosomal recessive mutation, or rapidly progressive severe to profound sensorineural with an autosomal dominant mutation [93-95].

5.1.2.6. *TMPRSS3*

TMPRSS3 codes for transmembrane protease serine 3, a protein whose function is unknown. Hearing loss can be congenital profound or postlingual progressive, often with a ski slope audiogram that eventually progresses to a flat loss [96, 97].

5.1.2.7. *TECTA*

TECTA codes for alpha tectorin, a major structural component of the tectorial membrane. Mutations in this gene are a common cause of mid-frequency hearing loss, exhibiting "notch" or "cookie-bite" audiograms. When inherited recessively, onset is either prelingual or postlingual during childhood or adolescence. (Autosomal dominant mutations are associated with a later age of onset.) Sensorineural hearing loss severity is moderate to profound, often with mid frequencies most affected, and may be progressive [98]. Mutations in this gene have been suggested to be associated with Jacobsen syndrome, a rare disorder characterized by developmental delays and abnormal blood clotting [99].

5.2. Nonsyndromic Hearing Loss: Autosomal Dominant Inheritance

Genes associated with autosomal dominant nonsyndromic hearing loss are responsible for a minority, though significant portion of cases. Again, there are too many genes for an exhaustive review. A brief description of the most common causative genes in autosomal dominant hearing loss follows.

5.2.1. WFS1

WFS1 codes for wolframin, a protein involved in ion homeostasis. Onset of hearing loss may be prelingual or postlingual in childhood or adolescence. It is characterized by a low-frequency sensorineural hearing loss. Frequencies up to 2 kHz are likely to be affected, but severity usually falls short of profound [100]. Tinnitus is a frequent complaint. Mutations in this gene also cause Wolfram syndrome. Wolfram syndrome is extremely rare and affects many systems. Deafness, progressive vision loss, diabetes mellitus, and diabetes insipidus are characteristic features [101].

5.2.2. KCNQ4

KCNQ4, also known as potassium voltage-gated channel, is another protein involved in ion homeostasis. Onset of hearing loss is postlingual, commonly in childhood to young adulthood. Hearing loss is sensorineural, with high frequencies affected first and mid to low frequencies affected later [102, 103]. Severity usually presents as mild to moderate and later progresses to profound. Around 25 to 35% of patients have an increased vestibulo-ocular reflex [104].

5.2.3. COCH

The *COCH* gene codes for cochlin, an extracellular matrix protein. Hearing loss tends to present in adulthood, and is progressive sensorineural, with high frequencies most affected. Aside from the hearing loss configuration, clinical presentation often closely mimics Meniere's disease. Vertigo, tinnitus, and aural fullness are all common complaints. Oculomotor disturbances are also common [105, 106].

5.2.4. GJB2

GJB2 codes for connexin 26, as previously discussed in section 5.1.1. This is the most common gene associated with autosomal recessive nonsyndromic hearing loss, but there are also mutations in this gene that cause autosomal dominant hearing loss. Onset of hearing loss may be later than the autosomal recessive variety, but often is prelingual or childhood-onset. Sensorineural hearing loss frequently begins in the high frequencies and progresses to affect the mid frequencies. In about half of cases, skin disorders are present, characterized by hyperkeratotic skin lesions [107]. The *GJB6* gene, also known as connexin 30, is a less common autosomal dominant hearing loss gene which shows a similar presentation, absent the skin lesions.

5.3. Nonsyndromic Hearing Loss: X-Linked Inheritance

X-linked nonsyndromic hearing loss is rare. The best-known gene in X-linked nonsyndromic hearing loss is *POU3F4*. Onset is prelingual. Mutations in this gene lead to defects in the bony labyrinth. Stapes fixation is common, and thus hearing loss may be mixed or sensorineural [108]. The stapes fixation may be addressed surgically, but there is a risk of perilymphatic gusher during surgery. Perilymphatic gusher is a phenomenon whereby a rush of perilymph exits the cochlea during stapedotomy or stapedectomy [109]. Because of this risk it is very helpful for the surgeon to know in advance of *POU3F4* involvement, both for risk assessment and surgery strategy. As with other X-linked genes, most affected individuals are male.

5.4. Nonsyndromic Hearing Loss: Mitochondrial Inheritance

Hearing loss due to a mutation in a mitochondrial gene is rare, but they are noteworthy because of their role in ototoxic-induced hearing loss. Recall from section 3.4 that mitochondria have their own genome separate from the nuclear genome. The mitochondrial genome consists of only 37 genes. A1555G is a mitochondrial mutation in the 12S rRNA gene, and it is the most common mitochondrial mutation causing hearing loss [110].

Since this is a mitochondrial mutation, it is inherited from the mother. The carrier rate is highest in Asian populations [110-112]. About half of individuals with this mutation develop hearing loss, usually after age 30. However, hearing loss can occur much earlier if an individual with this mutation receives aminoglycoside antibiotics (amikacin, dihydrostreptomycin, gentamicin, kanamycin, neomycin, streptomycin, tobramycin). Though rarely encountered in the United States, deafness associated with this mutation is much more common in China. The combination of high carrier rates and overuse of antibiotics has increased the rates of deafness due to this mutation in China [111, 112]. Use of aminoglycoside antibiotics over non-aminoglycosides should be carefully considered and utilized only when the benefits outweigh the risks.

The type of hearing loss is sensorineural. The degree of hearing loss can vary from mild to profound, but is likely to be severe to profound if the individual is exposed to aminoglycoside antibiotics. Hearing loss can occur a few days or weeks after aminoglycoside administration, even after a single dose [110]. As mitochondria are thought to have been independent single-celled organisms billions of years ago, their cellular structure and genome are similar to that of bacteria. Aminoglycoside antibiotics work by binding to the bacterial ribosome and disrupting protein function. The A1555G mutation essentially makes the ribosome more similar to a bacterial ribosome [113].

6. TECHNOLOGIES IN GENETIC TESTING

6.1. Cytogenetics

Cytogenetics is the branch of genetics that evaluates chromosome structure and function. This can be viewed as assessing the genome at the cellular level (cyto=cell). Visualizing chromosomes means we are "zoomed out" relative to molecular testing. The cellular view corresponds to a bird's-eye view: we are getting a large-scale view, but we cannot see small details. Cytogenetic testing is useful for detecting changes in chromosome number and structure: too many chromosomes, missing chromosomes, and large structural aberrations. It will not detect small rearrangements or mutations such as point mutations (substitution of one base of DNA for another). These rearrangements are simply too small for us to see from our zoomed-out vantage point. The major testing tools in cytogenetics are karyotyping, FISH, and array CGH. An explanation of each follows.

6.1.1. Classical Cytogenetics: Creation of a Karyotype

A karyotype is a preparation of chromosomes from one cell, in which the chromosomes are arranged according to their numerical assignments. Recall from section 2.3 that a human cell is expected to contain 46 chromosomes: 44 autosomes and 2 sex chromosomes. Males and females differ only in their sex chromosome complement. A typical male will have a karyotype of 46,XY and a typical female will have a karyotype of 46,XX. There are several steps necessary to prepare a karyotype. First, cells must be cultured anywhere from 24 hours to 8 to 10 days, depending on sample type and viability. Many sample types require addition of a mitogen, such as PHA (phytohemagglutinin) to stimulate cell division. Direct samples without culturing are sometimes used when results are needed urgently, but this is not utilized frequently, as morphology tends to be poor. Many different tissue types can be used for cytogenetic testing, including peripheral blood, bone marrow, amniotic fluid, chorionic villus sampling, skin biopsy, tumors, and products of conception (abortus material, typically from spontaneous abortions), among others. These tissue types represent the diverse patients who undergo cytogenetic testing. Diagnostic usefulness encompasses disparate needs, such as prenatal, cancer, developmental delay, and infertility. Buccal cells, epithelial cells collected through saliva or cheek swabs, cannot be used for cytogenetic testing because they do not grow sufficiently in culture. They can, however, be used in DNA testing (Sections 6.2 and 6.3).

After cells are cultured to increase cell growth and cell division, samples are harvested to obtain chromosome spreads which can be used in a karyotype. The purpose of the harvest procedure is to accumulate cells in metaphase of mitosis. This is the phase of mitosis where the chromosomes reach maximal condensation and are most readily analyzed. The harvest procedure requires a series of steps and takes several hours:

1. Incubation with colchicine: Colchicine poisons the mitotic spindle, which is necessary for chromosomes to split into two daughter cells and complete mitosis. Colchicine allows for a greater number of cells in culture to accumulate in metaphase. Without colchicine, very few cells would be in metaphase, making analysis difficult to impossible.
2. Incubation in a hypotonic solution: Cells are collected by centrifugation and a hypotonic solution is added. This solution will be at a concentration that is slightly hypotonic to the cells in culture. Through the property of osmosis, water will move from a less concentrated solution to a more concentrated solution. Water will therefore move from the hypotonic solution and into the cells. The purpose of this solution is to swell the cells just enough to allow the chromosomes to spread, but not enough so that the cells burst. Spreading the chromosomes aids greatly in analysis. Commonly used hypotonic solutions are potassium chloride and sodium citrate.
3. Addition of a fixative: After the appropriate incubation time in hypotonic solution, a fixative is added, typically a 3:1 solution of methanol:acetic acid. This fixes, or preserves the cells, and removes excess water and cellular debris. At this point the cells are no longer alive. Several fixative changes may be necessary.
4. Slide preparation: Cells are dropped onto slides and aged overnight on a hot plate.
5. Slide staining: Slides are treated with trypsin, an enzyme that digests proteins bound to DNA and allows the chromosomes to take up stain in a characteristic banding pattern. Slides are then stained with a deep stain, such as Giemsa or Wright stain.
6. Chromosome analysis and karyotyping: Chromosomes are analyzed under a light microscope at 100x magnification. An

imaging system attached to the microscope is used to photograph desired cells, which are then karyotyped on a computer. The end result is a completed karyotype (Figure 2).

For a more detailed review, see Howe et al. [114].

During chromosome analysis, the technologist will find a metaphase cell under the microscope suitable for analysis. The chromosomes are counted, and then evaluated one chromosome at a time to ensure all expected bands are present. For a typical case, 20 cells are analyzed. This may be increased to 50 or 100 cells if mosaicism is suspected or discovered. Mosaicism means that there is more than one chromosome complement in an individual. This is not common, but does sometimes occur due to a postzygotic nondisjunction event (see section 4.5).

Aside from chromosome number, cytogenetic analysis also seeks to discover structural aberrations. There are 4 major types of chromosome aberrations:

1. Deletion: A section of a chromosome is missing.
2. Duplication: A section of a chromosome is repeated.
3. Inversion: A section of a chromosome is flipped, as if a piece was removed, turned around, and then inserted back into the chromosome. With an inversion, no material is missing or gained, just rearranged. In most cases this is benign, such that the individual carrying a chromosomal inversion does not know unless they happen to get a karyotype. In rare cases an inversion can cause problems if the chromosome happens to be cut within a gene. A person carrying an inversion is also at increased risk of having a child with a deletion or duplication in the breakpoint regions.
4. Translocation: Sections of two or more chromosomes are exchanged with one another. Translocations can be balanced or unbalanced. When balanced, there is rarely a consequence to the individual carrying a translocation. However, like inversions, there is a risk to offspring because a child can inherit an unbalanced

form. When unbalanced, there will be extra material from one chromosome and missing material from another chromosome. This is essentially like having both a deletion and a duplication.

How deleterious these chromosomal aberrations are depends on several factors, and are not always predictable. In general, larger deletions and duplications are more deleterious than smaller ones, but very small deletions and duplications can have enormous consequences as well. The number of genes affected, redundancy of those genes, and influence of modifier genes will all affect the patient's clinical presentation. Chromosome analysis is useful for identifying these aberrations, but even the smallest deletions and duplications can only be visualized microscopically if they involve hundreds of thousands of base pairs of DNA. This is a major limitation of karyotyping. The next two techniques allow us to zoom in a bit further and identify smaller aberrations.

6.1.2. FISH: A Molecular Cytogenetic Technique

The smallest of chromosomal deletions that are visible microscopically are about 200 to 300 kilobases of DNA (1 kilobase=1,000 bases), and even that size is difficult unless chromosome length, spreading, and banding are optimal. These small deletions, also known as microdeletions, can be visualized by a technique known as FISH (fluorescence *in situ* hybridization). FISH is considered a molecular cytogenetic technique because it utilizes similar principles to that employed in polymerase chain reaction and other molecular techniques. The process is relatively simple. A slide is prepared after chromosome harvest, but the slide is not aged or stained. The slide is heated at high temperature to denature the DNA into two separate strands. A FISH probe is added to the slide and incubated. This probe consists of two components: a stretch of DNA (~100-300 kilobases) complementary in sequence to the desired area attached to a fluorophore. During incubation, the denatured DNA will renature with the FISH probe. The slide is visualized under a fluorescent microscope in the dark. The fluorophore present will excite and fluoresce when exposed to the appropriate wavelength of light. Fluorophores are available in a variety of colors, with red, green, and aqua being the most commonly used.

FISH has a few advantages over the karyotype. Its greatest advantage is in identifying microdeletions or microduplications that are too small to detect with standard cytogenetics. For most FISH probes, interphase cells can be analyzed, yielding many more cells to work with. Preparations by FISH also work fairly well on uncultured cells and the test has a fast turnaround time, making FISH more amenable to "stat" testing. A major drawback with FISH is that each probe used is only testing a very specific chromosomal region. In other words, you need to know what you are looking for. This usually means the physician must suspect the correct syndrome and request FISH testing for that syndrome. Figure 15 shows a picture of a cell tested with a FISH probe.

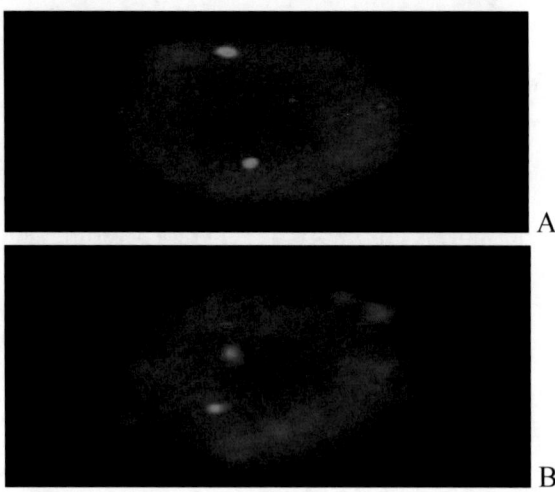

Figure 15. Fluorescence *in situ* hybridization (FISH). Pictures of human lymphocytes from two patients stained with FISH probes. These cells were probed for the *RB1* gene, a tumor suppressor gene located on chromosome 13, tagged with a red fluorescent probe. Deletion of *RB1* is associated with retinoblastoma, an aggressive ocular cancer. A centromere probe on chromosome 10, tagged with a green fluorescent probe, is used as a control. Since two copies of each *RB1* and chromosome 10 are expected, the anticipated result is two red signals and two green signals. The cell in A is normal, with two copies of each signal. The cell in B only has one red signal due to deletion of one copy of the *RB1* gene. This patient would be expected to develop retinoblastoma. FISH pictures are courtesy of the laboratory of Dr. Fern Tsien, Louisiana University Health Sciences Center Department of Genetics, used with permission.

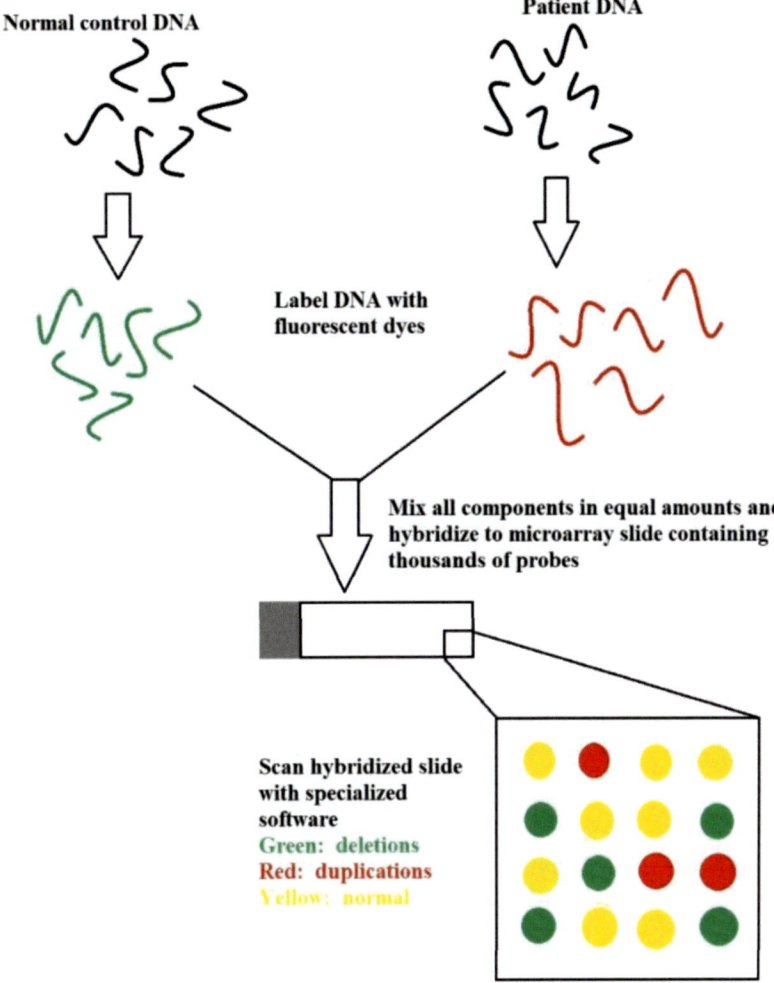

Figure 16. Array CGH. Array CGH (comparative genomic hybridization) is illustrated here. Thousands of probes are attached to a slide. DNA from the patient is mixed with normal control DNA and labeled with fluorescent dyes. After hybridization, the slide is scanned and analyzed with specialized software. The red and green dyes will appear yellow when combined in equal amounts. Areas of gene deletions will appear green (patient DNA is missing), while areas of gene duplications will appear red (patient DNA is in excess of control DNA). Balanced rearrangements are undetectable with this method.

6.1.3. Array CGH: Molecular Cytogenetics of the Entire Genome

In the last decade, the karyotype has been largely replaced with array CGH (comparative genomic hybridization). Array CGH is a technique that combines important components of karyotyping and FISH. A simplified view of array CGH is demonstrated in Figure 16. A microarray is a slide containing thousands of probes covering the entire human genome. DNA from the patient's sample is isolated and labeled with a fluorescent dye (red in this example). DNA from a known genetically normal individual of the same gender is labeled with a different fluorescent dye (green). The samples are mixed together and applied to the microarray, where they are incubated and allowed to hybridize to the thousands of probes on the array. The microarray slide is scanned by a computer with specialized software. Deletions and duplications are identified based on the color of every probe in the array. If there is no gain or loss of material, the color will appear yellow due to the mixing of the red and green probes. A loss of material (deletion) will appear green and a gain of material (duplication) will appear red. When a deletion or duplication is identified, it is confirmed by FISH testing.

Array CGH has many of the advantages of FISH probes, but the whole genome is evaluated much as in the karyotype. With this technique, it is not necessary to know exactly what you are looking for because all of the probes are already included. There is a major limitation of array CGH compared to karyotyping. Array CGH only shows gains and losses of genetic material. It will not show balanced rearrangements. Therefore, an individual carrying a balanced translocation or inversion will not be detected by array CGH. It is for this reason that the karyotype will not be completely supplanted by array CGH.

6.2. Polymerase Chain Reaction and Gel Electrophoresis

The polymerase chain reaction (better known as PCR) is perhaps the most significant advancement in molecular biology. Developed by Kary Mullis in 1983, PCR has revolutionized molecular genetics, being widely used in medicine, forensics, and scientific research. PCR is a method of amplifying DNA. This allows one to analyze a particular region of DNA when there are very small quantities present. The amplification of DNA is analogous to photocopying a page from a large book, as if that page was torn out and photocopied millions of times. PCR reactions are generally 30 to 100 μl in volume, but can be as low as 10 μl. Small quantities of the following are transferred by micropipet into PCR tubes:

1. DNA template: DNA from the sample to be tested
2. Primers: 2 short DNA sequences (~15-25 bases) complementary to the region/gene being tested
3. dNTPs (deoxynucleotide triphosphates): nucleotide bases A, G, C, T of DNA
4. DNA polymerase: enzyme that makes new DNA through addition of bases
5. Magnesium ions: works as a cofactor for DNA polymerase
6. Buffer solution: for stability of DNA polymerase.

The prepared PCR reactions are placed in a thermal cycler. A thermal cycler is a machine capable of rapidly changing temperature. This is the key to the PCR process, the bulk of which involves repeated cycles of short incubations at three different temperatures. First, the samples are heated to a high temperature around 95°C to denature the DNA sample. Once denatured, the temperature is quickly lowered to around 60°C, a temperature ideal for annealing. Annealing is where the primers bind to their complementary sequence of DNA. The temperature is then raised to 72°C for elongation, a temperature at which the polymerase enzyme works optimally. The polymerase adds bases from the dNTP mix. The polymerase used in PCR is *Taq* polymerase, obtained from the bacteria *Thermus aquaticus*. This species of bacteria thrives in very hot environments, and thus its polymerase is stable at very high temperatures. At the end of each PCR cycle, there are twice as many DNA fragments of the desired region. After 30 to 40 cycles of PCR, you are left with millions of copies of this DNA fragment, even if you started with just one. Figure 17 shows a simplified schematic diagram of this process.

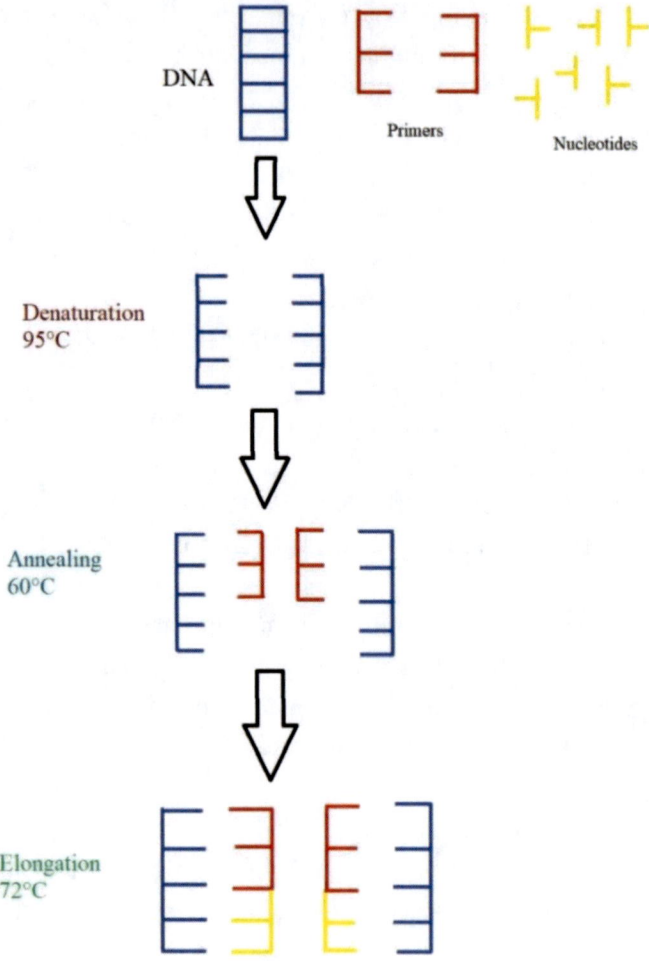

Figure 17. Polymerase Chain Reaction (PCR). One cycle of PCR is illustrated here. The DNA sample being tested is mixed with nucleotides and primers which will form the building blocks necessary to produce more DNA copies of a desired region of DNA. One cycle consists of denaturation, annealing, and elongation. The DNA is denatured into two strands by heating at a high temperature. The temperature is lowered to allow the primers to anneal to their complementary strands. The temperature is raised back up to the optimal working temperature of DNA polymerase, which will add nucleotides to build a new DNA strand. At the end of the PCR cycle, you are left with double the amount of DNA from the start of the cycle. A typical PCR run will include 30 to 40 cycles, resulting in millions of DNA copies of the desired gene or region. The PCR products can then be visualized via gel electrophoresis.

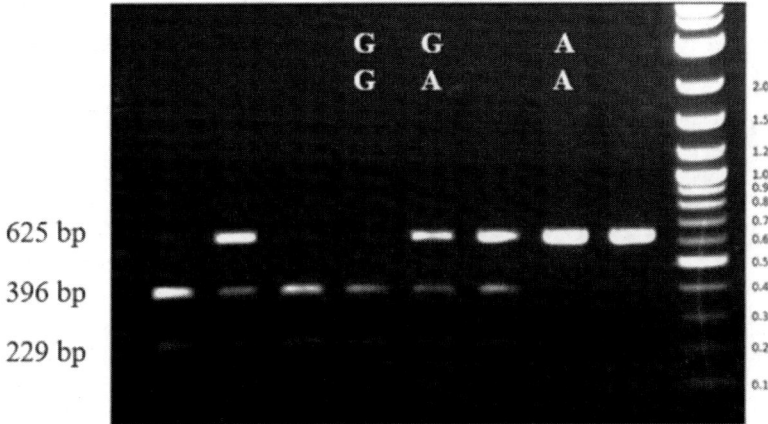

Figure 18. Gel electrophoresis. Agarose gel electrophoresis after PCR for the G216A mutation in the *USH1C* gene. The normal genotype at this site is GG. A substitution of G to A results in Usher syndrome if two copies are present (Usher syndrome is autosomal recessive). PCR products are separated by size, with smaller fragments moving faster through the gel. Fragment sizes in base pairs (bp) are listed on the left of the picture. The far right lane contains a DNA ladder of known fragment sizes. Three patient samples are labeled: GG (normal), GA (carrier for Usher syndrome), and AA (Usher syndrome). Gel picture courtesy of the laboratory of Dr. Fern Tsien, Louisiana University Health Sciences Center Department of Genetics, used with permission.

The PCR products can be loaded on a gel and run through gel electrophoresis to visualize the results. The main types of gels used are agarose and acrylamide. The gels are of a somewhat porous material so the DNA can move through the gel. An electric current is run through the gel after the samples are loaded. Since DNA has a negative charge, the samples are loaded at the negative pole and migrate toward the positive pole once the electric current is introduced. The gel acts as a sieve, allowing smaller DNA fragments to migrate through the gel at a faster rate than the larger fragments. The end result is a separation of DNA fragments based on size. A chemical dye such as ethidium bromide is added to the gel to allow for visualization. Ethidium bromide binds to DNA and fluoresces under ultraviolet light. An example of an agarose gel electrophoresis following PCR is shown in Figure 18.

PCR is specific and, if designed properly, can identify single base-pair changes. It is relatively cheap to run and has a great deal of versatility.

There are many downstream applications for PCR which are too complex to describe here. It can be regarded as a "zoomed-in" procedure. We are evaluating specifically what we designed our primers for, not the entire genome. We will therefore not identify a disorder in a different gene.

6.3. DNA Sequencing

DNA sequencing determines the exact base sequence of a strand of DNA. This can be a targeted sequencing or a whole genome sequencing. Targeted sequencing tests a specific region, usually a particular gene or set of genes. Whole genome sequencing tests the entire genome of an individual. The latter is obviously far more complex, time-consuming, and expensive. Major methods of DNA sequencing employed today are Sanger sequencing and next generation sequencing. Sanger sequencing was one of the original DNA sequencing techniques developed, and has largely been replaced by next generation sequencing techniques in the last decade. However, Sanger sequencing is still used, mostly for targeted sequencing. The process of DNA sequencing will not be discussed here. The interested reader is encouraged to explore this topic independently.

6.3.1. Genome Sequencing

In 1990, the Human Genome Project was launched as an international collaborative effort to sequence the entire human genome. It took years to complete, but finished ahead of schedule in 2003. Today's next generation sequencing techniques have managed to drastically cut down the testing time. In recent years, whole genome sequencing is gaining widespread use in clinical testing. It has become cheaper and faster, and has allowed for a diagnosis in patients who previously tested normal by other methods. However, it is still expensive relative to other methods, and turnaround time by a clinical laboratory takes several weeks or months for testing and analysis of results. Exome sequencing is a frequently-used alternative that cuts down on the amount of DNA to analyze.

6.3.2. Exome Sequencing

Over 98% of the human genome does not code for proteins. When performing clinical testing on a patient suspected of a genetic disorder, sequencing analysis can be greatly reduced by focusing on these coding regions. Recall from section 2.1 that genes are transcribed into mRNA. The initial mRNA is a complement to the DNA gene from which it was transcribed. Human genes contain exons and introns. Exons are the sequences responsible for coding for the resultant protein, while introns contain regulatory elements and non-coding sequences. The evolutionary purpose of introns is unclear. As the introns are unnecessary for coding of the protein, they are removed from the mature mRNA molecule. This is illustrated in Figure 19. The exons now can be sequenced without the baggage of the introns. This process is exome sequencing. It has the advantage over whole genome sequencing of being cheaper and faster while still having the capability of finding most of the same mutations. However, while uncommon, deleterious intronic mutations do exist. An intronic mutation can affect a regulatory element, which can cause the exons to be spliced in an alternative way. This can affect the protein product and cause disease. Exome sequencing will not identify all intronic mutations.

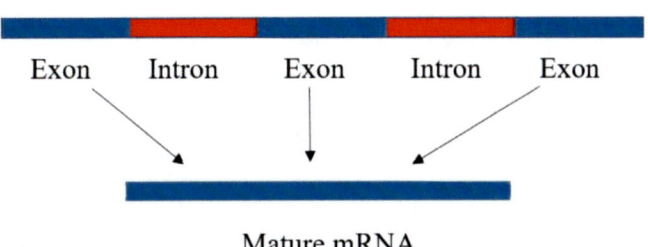

Figure 19. Exons and introns. The DNA sequence of a gene includes exons (coding regions) and introns (noncoding regions). Once a DNA sequence is transcribed into mRNA, the introns are removed and the exons are joined together during a process known as RNA splicing. Exome sequencing analyzes only the exons. Most disease-causing mutations will be found in the exons, and thus exome sequencing is a quicker and more cost-effective method for identifying mutations. However, deleterious mutations do occur on occasion in the introns if they lead to aberrant splicing. Genomic sequencing analyzes both exons and introns.

While genome and exome sequencing are not yet mainstream clinical applications for testing patients with nonsyndromic hearing loss, they are being used in research settings. This is leading to identification of more genes associated with hearing loss. As the cost continues to drop these tests may gain traction for diagnosis of genetic hearing loss.

7. MAKING A GENETICS REFERRAL

7.1. When Should a Genetics Referral Be Made?

For most patients who may benefit from genetic testing, a referral from a health care professional is needed, as few patients or families will seek this out themselves. In cases of hearing loss with a genetic etiology, the audiologist is a key player in achieving this diagnosis. Of course, any health care professional can recommend a genetics evaluation, and this is frequently initiated by primary care physicians and specialty physicians. However, in cases of hearing loss, physicians may defer to audiologists to make these calls. On the other hand, audiologists frequently defer to physicians to address genetic testing because the evaluation is viewed as medical in nature. Unfortunately, this results in many patients being missed until other health effects from a syndrome surface or hearing loss recurs in another family member. By this time many of the benefits of genetic testing have been lost. If audiologists want to be viewed as the authority on hearing loss, we must take a leadership role in all aspects of hearing and balance, including genetics of hearing loss. This is particularly applicable to pediatric audiologists, whose patients and families have the most to gain from a genetics evaluation. Deferring the referral to physicians, many of whom know far less about both hearing loss and genetics than audiologists, we are missing an opportunity to assert our expertise. This ultimately results in a disservice to our patients. This does not mean that every audiologist must be an expert in genetics or have an in-depth understanding of genes involved in hearing loss or genetic testing methods. It does mean, however, that every audiologist should understand when to make a genetics referral, how to talk to patients and families about genetic testing, and what the ramifications are of various test results. (For clarification, the use of the term *referral* in this chapter is roughly equivalent to *recommendation*. It is not used in association with insurance coverage, which varies by plan and may require a physician order. Insurance coverage is inconsistent for genetic testing.)

So when should an audiologist make a referral for a genetics evaluation? Put simply, a referral can be made in any case of permanent hearing loss with an unknown etiology if the patient or family desires. This will start with a discussion with the patient or the patient's family (in pediatric cases) about the possibility of a genetic etiology. This should be done in a sensitive manner, and may begin by asking if they have ever considered genetic testing or a genetic etiology. This will help assess whether anyone else has suggested a genetic etiology and what the family thinks about it. This can begin the conversation and allow the audiologist to discuss possible benefits of receiving a genetics evaluation. It should be noted that genetic testing is not for everyone, and it will not benefit everyone. Some patients and families will elect to decline a genetics referral for a variety of reasons. This is their choice and that choice should be respected. Patients and families should never feel pressured to undergo genetic testing or shamed for declining. Our role as audiologists is to ensure patients are made aware of the possibility of a genetic etiology and have the opportunity to seek that out should they desire. Patients should also be made aware that an evaluation with a geneticist and/or genetic counselor does not mean they will or must receive genetic testing. Part of this evaluation should include assessment for emotional readiness for genetic testing, which may conclude with declination of testing.

There are several characteristics which, when present, increase the likelihood of a genetic etiology, and should therefore be considered when discussing a genetics referral. Perhaps the strongest is a family history of hearing loss, particularly a family history of congenital or early-onset hearing loss. An increase in the number of relatives and closeness of relationship with the patient will each increase the likelihood that the cause is genetic. First-degree relatives (children, parents, and siblings) carry the most weight because these relatives share, on average, half of their DNA with one another (or all of their DNA, in the case of monozygotic twins). Second-degree relatives (aunts, uncles, grandparents) share, on average, a quarter of their DNA, and are also significant in the family history. Third-degree relatives (such as first cousins) should not be dismissed, especially if there are two or more affected family members. Third-degree relatives carry greater weight in families with consanguinity, meaning there is a mating between blood relatives. In families with consanguinity there is an increased risk of having offspring with an autosomal recessive disorder. This may include deafness/hearing loss. While a family history of hearing loss increases the chances of a genetic etiology, the absence of a family history does not exclude a genetic cause. Recall that over 90% of children born with permanent hearing loss are born to hearing parents, and in many cases there is no known family history on either side. Genetics referrals should not be dismissed because there is no family history. The Joint Committee on Infant Hearing position statement recommends referral for a genetics evaluation for children born with permanent hearing loss [115].

Another characteristic increasing the likelihood of a genetic etiology is the presence of other clinical features. These features may be readily apparent, such as dysmorphologies or distinct facial features, or they may be less conspicuous. Hearing loss accompanied by cardiac problems, kidney problems, thyroid problems, vision loss, fainting spells, or skin lesions should be heavily suspected as being genetic. In addition, hearing loss (especially deafness) occurring after administration of a normal dose of aminoglycoside antibiotics may be due to a genetic mutation. If common hearing loss-associated infections have been ruled out as the cause, odds are increased that the cause is genetic. Finally, unusual audiometric configurations (such as "cookie-bite" audiograms or low-frequency sensorineural hearing loss) often have a genetic cause, especially if there is a family history.

Most genetics referrals are made for pediatric patients or cases where a syndrome is suspected. These are the patients and families who have the most to gain from genetic testing. In cases of adult-onset nonsyndromic hearing loss, a referral may or may not be made. For many of these patients the costs may outweigh the benefits. Nonetheless, a discussion could be held with the patient, and a referral considered in the presence of a strong family history if the patient desires. In the absence of a strong family history in a patient with adult-onset hearing loss, genetic testing is unlikely to yield useful information. Genetic testing can be laborious, expensive, and emotionally draining, and it is not always fruitful. Benefits, impacts, and limitations of genetic testing must all be considered with each patient. This will be the responsibility of clinical geneticists and genetic counselors.

7.2. Benefits of Genetic Testing

There are several potential benefits of genetic testing for patients with hearing loss. In cases of syndromic hearing loss, the diagnosis can direct clinical evaluation and treatment for associated disorders. For example, a diagnosis of Jervell and Lange-Nielsen syndrome will lead to close monitoring for cardiac issues. Without this diagnosis, the patient would not know to seek treatment until experiencing an adverse event. Likewise, a diagnosis of Usher syndrome received before the onset of vision loss would allow for the patient to undergo ophthalmologic evaluation and the patient's family to prepare for the future, such as early teaching of Braille. Patients have a better opportunity to take care of themselves if they are aware of potential health consequences associated with their syndrome.

Another major benefit of genetic testing is an allowance of estimation of recurrence risks for patients and/or their families. For some families this will be very important and may be the driving motivation for obtaining genetic testing. For other families, this will not be important at all. Discussions on recurrence risks, handled by the genetics team, should be addressed sensitively. It should not be assumed that all families will want this information, and some may feel offended by the topic. However, there will be families who would like to know the odds of having another affected child, and they may or may not use this information for family-planning purposes.

A genetic diagnosis may affect distant members of the patient's family, should the family opt to share this information. Depending on the family, this may be viewed as a benefit, a drawback, or of no consequence. If other family members are informed of the diagnosis, this may enable them to receive an early diagnosis, thereby optimizing treatment and yielding risk estimates for their offspring. However, distant family members may not welcome this information, and may even be resentful that it is thrust upon them. On the other hand, some families may not want to share their diagnosis with family members, either because they are not close to their family, they want to keep their medical information private, or they are unsure if the information will be welcome. These different scenarios may cause tension amongst family members or feelings of guilt in members of the presenting family.

In some cases there may be no real benefit other than having a diagnosis. For some families it is satisfying to know the reason behind the hearing loss and other features (if present) even if it is of no consequence in family-planning or health monitoring. Some patients or parents find peace of mind in knowing the cause, which can be a benefit in and of itself. The benefits of genetic testing are less clear with adult-onset hearing loss. By adulthood, a syndrome likely would have been identified already, and recurrence risks are usually not important to individuals who may pass on adult-onset hearing loss. Also, by the time someone reaches adulthood there are many other potential causes to consider, lowering the chances of identifying a genetic etiology. Nonetheless, there may be patients where testing may be pursued. Again, genetic testing for these patients is often futile unless there are several family members affected with a similar presentation (i.e., type, onset, progression, and configuration of hearing loss).

7.3. Impacts of a Positive Genetic Test Result

During the genetics evaluation, the genetic counselor will discuss with the patient and/or patient's family how they may be impacted by the results of the test. This will be taken into consideration before genetic testing is performed. A positive test result can have negative psychological or social effects for the patient and the patient's family. Genes make up who we are, causing a genetic diagnosis to feel deeply personal for some people. As previously discussed, a positive test result can affect other family members who may or may not be prepared to receive this information. For parents, feelings of guilt are common. Tension between parents may ensue, especially if the mutation in question is found to be inherited exclusively from one parent. Parents may be prone to assign blame, even if inadvertently. Some have raised ethical concerns with the genetic testing of children, arguing such testing violates a child's right not to know. There is legitimacy to this argument; genetic testing of minor children should never be taken lightly. These issues should be explored with the genetic counselor when the family is deciding whether or not to pursue genetic testing.

7.4. Limitations of Genetic Testing

Just as there are potential ramifications to patients and their families with a positive test result, families must also face the possibility of a negative test result. Families may complete genetic testing feeling lost and confused if the process does not result in a diagnosis. This outcome is far more common than one might expect when considering the prevalence of genetic hearing loss, and there are a few reasons why this would happen. The most obvious explanation for a negative test result is that the cause of the hearing loss is not genetic. However, one cannot conclude this based on a negative genetic test result unless there is another viable explanation for the etiology, in which case genetic testing probably would never have been initiated. This may be the most common error made by patients and health care providers alike regarding genetic test results. On the contrary, a negative result on a genetic test does not necessarily mean the cause is not genetic. Rather, one can only conclude that a genetic etiology for what the test examined can be ruled out.

Recall that there are over 400 genes associated with syndromic hearing loss and over 100 genes associated with nonsyndromic hearing loss. Consider a patient with nonsyndromic congenital deafness with an extensive family history presents for genetic testing. Based on evaluation of family history of autosomal recessive inheritance and limited insurance coverage for genetic testing, a decision is made to sequence the patient's *GJB2* gene, also known as connexin 26. Because mutations in connexin 26 cause more cases of nonsyndromic hearing loss than any other gene, this approach is reasonable. Testing comes back as negative and this is reported to the family. All that can be concluded from this result is that connexin 26 is not the cause of deafness in this patient (and presumably in this family, although some families have been found to have more than one causative gene). We have no information on the 100+ other genes which were not tested. If a result is still desired, another gene must be selected for testing, and it is not easy deciding which way to go next. To make this example even more specific, let us imagine that instead of sequencing connexin 26, a molecular test is performed for 35delG, the most common mutation in connexin 26 deafness. The test may be ordered this way because it is even more cost-effective than sequencing of the entire gene, but it will only detect cases caused by the 35delG mutation. In this example, a negative result would not even rule out connexin 26 as the causative gene. Rather, it would only rule out a connexin 26 35delG mutation.

Because testing is expensive and insurance companies will not always cover it, starting with the most likely gene to yield a positive result is a common approach. Over the last decade gene panels for various disorders, including hearing loss have been developed. Hearing loss panels are offered by some testing laboratories, and allow for simultaneous molecular testing of many mutations in several different genes, increasing the likelihood of a positive result in a single test. Sequencing tests will identify more mutations, but the time and costs involved make it prohibitive for many patients, especially in cases of nonsyndromic hearing loss. Fortunately, these comprehensive tests have been getting gradually faster and cheaper, so they may be more accessible for clinical testing in the future. However, even sequencing does not identify the causative gene for all patients. Exome sequencing only sequences the coding regions of genes, which is where most mutations occur. But mutations in introns can disrupt regulatory elements in genes, affecting gene expression. Sequencing the entire genome will include intronic regions, but the large amount of data generated can be difficult to interpret. Thus, sequencing can miss the cause because the gene in question has not been identified to be associated with the disorder being tested. As testing methods improve there will be fewer patients who do not obtain a diagnosis. But in today's world, a negative test result is common for families of hearing loss as well as many genetic disorders.

7.5. Testing Recommendations

The testing panel will be determined by the geneticist. Audiologists can aid the process by communicating pertinent information about the patient's audiological evaluation [116]. This includes type of hearing loss, severity, age of onset, progression, audiometric configuration, family history, and presence of auditory neuropathy or vestibular disturbance. These characteristics can give clues on which gene may be involved. If audiograms are available from affected family members, these may prove to be helpful as well. In cases of nonsyndromic hearing loss, the presenting characteristics may be suggestive of inheritance pattern. Nonsyndromic hearing loss with an autosomal recessive inheritance pattern is more likely to have a prelingual onset, be stable in degree, and affect most or all frequencies. Conversely, nonsyndromic hearing loss with an autosomal dominant inheritance pattern is more likely to have a postlingual onset, be progressive, and affect a subset of frequencies. These are *general* characteristics, and vary by gene, mutation, individual, and family. They will *not* always hold true, but should be considered in conjunction with the inheritance pattern displayed in the family history. Due to the high incidence of congenital and early-onset hearing loss caused by cytomegalovirus (CMV), this infection should be considered when reviewing a patient's medical history. Newborn screening for CMV is being tested in hospitals in the United States, and may be incorporated in the future as part of the newborn hearing screening program [117]. CMV-related hearing loss presentation can appear similar to genetic hearing loss. A positive CMV test will prevent unnecessary genetic testing. Unfortunately, CMV testing methods lack sensitivity to reliably detect congenital CMV after 3 weeks of age [117]. This topic is sure to receive a great deal of attention in the years to come.

If the patient exhibits dysmorphic features along with hearing loss, testing may begin with array CGH followed by exome sequencing if the array CGH test is negative. If the geneticist suspects a specific syndrome, a molecular test specific for that syndrome may be ordered. This may involve a panel if it is a syndrome with multiple causative genes. Molecular tests for a specific syndrome are generally more cost-effective than sequencing techniques, but if results continue to be negative, exome sequencing may be warranted. A diagnosis is invaluable for patients who have significant health problems.

Once all tests have been exhausted, a negative result can be discouraging for a patient who stands to benefit from a genetic diagnosis. For these patients, audiologists may revisit the topic every 3 to 5 years and suggest a new genetics evaluation. Testing methods evolve quickly. A patient who received a negative result a few years ago may now be eligible for a test that either was not available previously or was too expensive. If the patient or the family still desires and could benefit from a genetic diagnosis this may be welcomed.

CONCLUSION

Audiologists are central figures in the health care teams treating patients with hearing loss. Since as many as 75-80% of early-onset permanent hearing losses are genetic and most adult-onset permanent hearing losses probably have a genetic component, it is imperative audiologists have a basic understanding of genetics if we are to fully serve our patients. Audiologists need not be genetics experts, but should understand when a genetics referral should be proposed and should be comfortable discussing this topic with their patients. Genetic testing has limitations and potential negative consequences which must be considered. The benefits of testing should outweigh the risks. If a patient is willing to complete a genetics evaluation, the geneticist and/or genetic counselor will determine if genetic testing is appropriate. To locate a genetic counselor, visit the National Society of Genetic Counselors at https://www.nsgc.org [118].

Completion of the Human Genome Project has allowed for the identification of thousands of genes, including many new genes found to be associated with deafness/hearing loss. As technology advances, more patients are able to receive a genetic diagnosis, and the tests continue to become faster, cheaper, and more sensitive. While new genes are sure to be linked to hearing loss in the future, genetic research is beginning to shift toward bioinformatics. Bioinformatics marries biology with computer science. Sophisticated software is used to analyze biological data and make predictions about their functions. This means that many research studies are moving out of the laboratory and onto the computer. Bioinformatics analyses may include predicting whether a gene mutation will cause deleterious protein function, predicting how a protein will fold, or examining how two different genes interact with one another. These studies will add new layers of complexity to our understanding of genes and how they function. In addition, our understanding of adult-onset hearing loss, to include presbycusis and noise-induced hearing loss, is bound to expand. Limited studies have suggested genetic determinants may influence our susceptibility to noise-induced hearing loss. It has been recognized for decades that individuals respond differently to noise exposure. Genetic polymorphisms or gene-environment interactions may help explain this phenomenon and could lead to noise protection recommendations customized for each individual. Likewise, presbycusis (age-related hearing loss), known to vary widely across the population, may have more to do with genetic differences than the aging process itself. The decades to come are sure to deliver exciting new discoveries in the world of genetic hearing loss.

REFERENCES

[1] National Institutes of Health. 2010. *Newborn hearing screening fact sheet.* Accessed December 24, 2018. https://report.nih.gov/NIH factsheets/ViewFactSheet.aspx?csid=104.

[2] Shargorodsky, J., Curhan, S.G., Curhan, G.C., and Eavey, R. 2010. "Change in prevalence of hearing loss in US adolescents." *JAMA* 304(7):772-778.

[3] Rehm, H.L. 2005. "A genetic approach to the child with sensorineural hearing loss." *Semin Perinatol* 29, 173-181.

[4] Smith, R.J., Bale, Jr., J.F., and White, K.R. 2005. "Sensorineural hearing loss in children." *Lancet* 365, 879-890.

[5] Shearer, A.E., Hildebrand, M.S., and Smith, R.J.H. 2017. "Hereditary hearing loss and deafness overview." In *Gene Reviews*, edited by M.P. Adam, H.H. Ardinger, R.A. Pagon, Wallace, S.E., Bean, L.J.H., Stephens, K., and Amemiya, A. Seattle, WA: University of Washington, Seattle Press. (PMID 20301607).

[6] Cohen, B.E., Durstenfeld, A., and Roehm, P.C. 2013. "Viral causes of hearing loss: a review for hearing health professionals." *Trends Hear* 18, 1-17.

[7] Ezkurdia, I., Juan, D., Rodriguez, J.M., Frankish, A., Diekhans, M., Harrow, J., Vazquez, J., Valencia, A., and Tress, M.L. 2014. "Multiple evidence strands suggest that there may be as few as 19,000 human protein-coding genes." *Hum Mol Genet* 23(22):5866-5878.

[8] Toriello, H.V., Reardon, W., and Gorlin, R.J. 2004. *Hereditary hearing loss and its syndromes.* New York: Oxford University Press.

[9] Van Camp, G., and Smith, R. 2018. *Hereditary Hearing Loss Homepage.* Accessed November 3, 2018. http://hereditaryhearing loss.org.

[10] Venter, J.C. et al. 2001. "The sequence of the human genome." *Science* 291(5507):1304-1351.

[11] Strachan, T., and Read, A.P. 1999. *Human molecular genetics.* New York: Wiley-Liss.

[12] Mitchell, R.E., and Karchmer, M.A. 2004. "Chasing the mythical ten percent: parental hearing status of deaf and hard of hearing students in the United States." *Sign Language Studies* 4(2):138-163.

[13] Robin, N.H., Moran, R.T., and Ala-Kokko, L. 2017. "Stickler syndrome." In *Gene Reviews*, edited by M.P. Adam, H.H. Ardinger, R.A. Pagon, Wallace, S.E., Bean, L.J.H., Stephens, K., and Amemiya, A. Seattle, WA: University of Washington, Seattle Press. (PMID 20301479).

[14] Acke, F.R., Dhooge, I.J., Malfait, F., and De Leenheer, E.M. 2012. "Hearing impairment in Stickler syndrome: a systematic review." *Orphanet J Rare Dis* 7:84. Accessed November 17, 2018. doi: 10.1186/1750-1172-7-84.

[15] Blake, K.D., and Prasad, C. 2006. "CHARGE syndrome." *Orphanet J Rare Dis* 1:34.

[16] Lalani, S.R., Hefner, M.A., Belmont, J.W., and Davenport, S.L.H. 2012. "CHARGE syndrome." In *Gene Reviews*, edited by M.P. Adam, H.H. Ardinger, R.A. Pagon, Wallace, S.E., Bean, L.J.H., Stephens, K., and Amemiya, A. Seattle, WA: University of Washington, Seattle Press. (PMID 20301296).

[17] Bergman, J.E., Janssen, N., Hoefsloot, L.H., Jongmans, M.C., Hofstra, R.M., van Ravenswaaij-Arts, C.M. 2011. "CHD7 mutations and CHARGE syndrome: the clinical implications of an expanding phenotype." *J Med Genet* 48(5):334-342.

[18] Hale, C.L., Niederriter, A.N., Green, G.E., and Martin, D.M. 2016. "Atypical phenotypes associated with pathogenic CHD7 variants and a proposal for broadening CHARGE syndrome clinical diagnostic criteria." *Am J Med Genet A* 170A(2):344-354.

[19] Sanlaville, D., Etchevers, H.C., Gonzales, M., Martinovic, J., Clement-Ziza, M., Delezoide, A.L., Aubry, M.C., Pelet, A., Chemouny, S., Cruaud, C., Audollent, S., Esculpavit, C., Goudefroye, G., Ozilou, C., Fredouille, C., Joye, N., Morichon-Delvallez, N., Dumez, Y., Weissenbach, J., Munnich, A., Amiel, J., Encha-Razavi, F., Lyonnet, S., Vekemans, M., and Attie-Bitach, T. 2006. "Phenotype spectrum of CHARGE syndrome in fetuses with

CHD7 truncating mutations correlates with expression during human development." *J Med Genet* 43(3):211-217.

[20] Zentner, G.E., Layman, W.S., Martin, D.M., and Scacheri, P.C. 2010. "Molecular and phenotypic aspects of CHD7 mutation in CHARGE syndrome." *Am J Med Genet A* 152A(3):674-686.

[21] Boyle, M.I., Jespersgaard, C., Brondum-Nielsen, K., Bisgaard, A.M., and Tumer, Z. 2015. "Cornelia de Lange syndrome." *Clin Genet* 88(1):1-12.

[22] Deardorff, M.A., Noon, S.E., and Krantz, I.D. 2016. "Cornelia de Lange syndrome." In *Gene Reviews*, edited by M.P. Adam, H.H. Ardinger, R.A. Pagon, Wallace, S.E., Bean, L.J.H., Stephens, K., and Amemiya, A. Seattle, WA: University of Washington, Seattle Press. (PMID 20301283).

[23] Deardorff, M.A., Bando, M., Nakato, R., Watrin, E., Itoh, T., Minamino, M., Saitoh, K., Komata, M., Katou, Y., Clark, D., Cole, K.E., De Baere, E., De Croos, C., Di Donato, N., Ernst, S., Francey, L.J., Gyftodimou, Y., Hirashima, K., Hullings, M., Ishikawa, Y., Jaulin, C., Kaur, M., Kiyono, T., Lombardi, P.M., Magnaghi-Jaulin, L., Mortier, G.R., Nozaki, N., Petersen, M.B., Seimiya, H., Siu, V.M., Suzuki, Y., Takagaki, K., Wilde, J.J., Willems, P.J., Prigent, C., Gillesen-Kaesbach, G., Christianson, D.W., Kaiser, F.J., Jackson, L.G., Hirota, T., Krantz, I.D., and Shirahige, K. 2012. "HDAC8 mutations in Cornelia de Lange syndrome affect the cohesin acetylation cycle." *Nature* 489(7415):313-317.

[24] Deardorff, M.A., Wilde, J.J., Albrecht, M., Dickinson, E., Tennstedt, S., Braunholz, D., Monnich, M., Yan, Y., Xu, W., Gil-Rodriguez, M.C., Clark, D., Hakonarson, H., Halbach, S., Michelis, L.D., Rampuria, A., Rossier, E., Spranger, S., Van Maldergem, L., Lynch, S.A., Gillesen-Kaesbach, G., Ludecke, H.J., Ramsay, R.G., McKay, M.J., Krantz, I.D., Xu, H., Horsfield, J.A., and Kaiser, F.J. 2012. "RAD21 mutations cause a human cohesinopathy." *Am J Hum Genet* 90(6):1014-1027.

[25] Krantz, I.D., McCallum, J., DeScipio, C., Kaur, M., Gillis, L.A., Yaeger, D., Jukofsky, L., Wasserman, N., Bottani, A., Morris, C.A.,

Nowaczyk, M.J., Toriello, H., Bamshad, M.J., Carey, J.C., Rappaport, E., Kawauchi, S., Lander, A.D., Calof, A.L., Li, H.H., Devoto, M., and Jackson, L.G. 2004. "Cornelia de Lange syndrome is caused by mutations in NIPBL, the human homolog of Drosophila melanogaster Nipped-B." *Nat Genet* 36(6):631-635.

[26] Tonkin, E.T., Wang, T.J., Lisgo, S., Bamshad, M.J., and Strachan, T. 2004. "NIPBL, encoding a homolog of fungal Scc2-type sister chromatid cohesion proteins and fly Nipped-B, is mutated in Cornelia de Lange syndrome." *Nat Genet* 36(6):636-641.

[27] Asthagiri, A.R., Parry, D.M., Butman, J.A., Kim, H.J., Tsilou, E.T., Zhuang, Z., and Lonser, R.R. 2009. "Neurofibromatosis type 2." *Lancet* 373(9679):1974-1986.

[28] Evans, D.G. 2018. "Neurofibromatosis 2." In *Gene Reviews*, edited by M.P. Adam, H.H. Ardinger, R.A. Pagon, Wallace, S.E., Bean, L.J.H., Stephens, K., and Amemiya, A. Seattle, WA: University of Washington, Seattle Press. (PMID 20301380).

[29] Shannon, R.V. 2011. "Auditory brainstem implants." *The ASHA Leader.* Accessed December 28, 2018. https://leader.pubs.asha.org/doi/10.1044/leader.FTR3sb3.16032011.17

[30] Evans, D.G. 2009. "Neurofibromatosis type 2 (NF2): a clinical and molecular review." *Orphanet J Rare Dis* 4:16. Accessed November 18, 2018. doi:10.1186/1750-1172-4-16.

[31] Kochhar, A., Fischer, S.M., Kimberling, W.J., and Smith, R.J. 2007. "Branchio-oto-renal syndrome." *Am J Med Genet A* 143A(14):1671-1678.

[32] Smith, R.J.H. 2018. "Branchiootorenal spectrum disorder." In *Gene Reviews*, edited by M.P. Adam, H.H. Ardinger, R.A. Pagon, Wallace, S.E., Bean, L.J.H., Stephens, K., and Amemiya, A. Seattle, WA: University of Washington, Seattle Press. (PMID 20301554).

[33] Fraser, F.C., Sproule, J.R., and Halal, F. 1980. "Frequency of the branchio-oto-renal (BOR) syndrome in children with profound hearing loss." *Am J Med Genet* 7:341-349.

[34] Chang, E.H., Menezes, M., Meyer, N.C., Cucci, R.A., Vervoort, V.S., Schwartz, C.E., and Smith, R.J. 2004. "Branchio-oto-renal

syndrome: the mutation spectrum in EYA1 and its phenotypic consequences." *Hum Mutat* 23(6):582-589.

[35] Hoskins, B.E., Cramer, C.H., Silvius, D., Zou, D., Raymond, R.M., Orten, D.J., Kimberling, W.J., Smith, R.J., Weil, D., Petit, C., Otto, E.A., Xu, P.X., and Hildebrandt, F. 2007. "Transcription factor SIX5 is mutated in patients with branchio-oto-renal syndrome." *Am J Hum Genet* 80(4):800-804.

[36] Orten, D.J., Fischer, S.M., Sorensen, J.L., Radhakrishna, U., Cremers, C.W., Marres, H.A., Van Camp, G., Welch, K.O., Smith, R.J., and Kimberling, W.J. 2008. "Branchio-oto-renal syndrome (BOR): novel mutations in the EYA1 gene, and a review of the mutational genetics of BOR." *Hum Mutat* 29(4):537- 544.

[37] Genetics Home Reference. 2018. *Branchiootorenal/branchiootic syndrome.* Accessed November 10, 2018. https://ghr.nlm.nih.gov/condition/branchiootorenal-branchiootic-syndrome#inheritance

[38] de Sousa Andrade, S.M., Monteiro, A.R., Martins, J.H., Alves, M.C., Santos Silva, L.F., Quadros, J.M., and Ribeiro, C.A. 2012. "Cochlear implant rehabilitation outcomes in Waardenburg syndrome children." *Int J Pediatr Otorhinolaryngol* 76, 1375-1378.

[39] Read, A.P., and Newton, V.E. 1997. "Waardenburg syndrome." *J Med Genet* 34, 656-665.

[40] Newton, V. 1990. "Hearing loss and Waardenburg syndrome: implications for genetic counseling." *J Laryngol Otol* 104, 97-103.

[41] Pardono, E., van Bever, Y., van den Ende, J., Havrenne, P.C., Iughetti, P., Maestrelli, S.R., Costa, F.O., Richieri-Costa, A., Frota-Pessoa, O., and Otto, P.A. 2003. "Waardenburg syndrome: clinical differentiation between types I and II." *Am J Med Genet A* 117A(3):223-235.

[42] Pingault, V., Ente, D., Dastot-Le Moal, F., Goossens, M., Marlin, S., and Bondurand, N. 2010. "Review and update of mutations causing Waardenburg syndrome." *Hum Mutat* 31(4):391-406.

[43] National Center for Biotechnology Information. 2018. *OMIM-Online Mendelian Inheritance in Man.* Johns Hopkins University. Accessed December 23, 2018. https://www.omim.org/

[44] Marszalek, B., Wojcicki, P., Kobus, K., and Trzeciak, W.H. 2002. "Clinical features, treatment and genetic background of Treacher Collins syndrome." *J Appl Genet* 43(2):223-233.

[45] Posnick, J.C., and Ruiz, R.L. 2000. "Treacher Collins syndrome: current evaluation, treatment, and future directions." *Cleft Palate Craniofac J* 37(5):434.

[46] Katsanis, S.H., and Jabs, E.W. 2018. "Treacher Collins syndrome." In *Gene Reviews*, edited by M.P. Adam, H.H. Ardinger, R.A. Pagon, Wallace, S.E., Bean, L.J.H., Stephens, K., and Amemiya, A. Seattle, WA: University of Washington, Seattle Press. (PMID 20301704).

[47] Sakai, D., and Trainor, P.A. 2009. "Treacher Collins syndrome: unmasking the role of Tcof1/treacle." *Int J Biochem Cell Biol* 41(6):1229-1232.

[48] Dixon, J., and Dixon, M.J. 2004. "Genetic background has a major effect on the penetrance and severity of craniofacial defects in mice heterozygous for the gene encoding the nuclear protein Treacle." *Dev Dyn* 229, 907-914.

[49] Carinci, F., Pezzetti, F., Locci, P., Becchetti, E., Carls, F., Avantaggiato, A., Becchetti, A., Carinci, P., Baroni, T., and Bodo, M. 2005. "Apert and Crouzon syndromes: clinical findings, genes and extracellular matrix." *J Craniofac Surg* 16(3):361-368.

[50] Robin, N.H., Falk, M.J., and Haldeman-Englert, C.R. 2011. "FGFR-related craniosynostosis syndromes." In *Gene Reviews*, edited by M.P. Adam, H.H. Ardinger, R.A. Pagon, Wallace, S.E., Bean, L.J.H., Stephens, K., and Amemiya, A. Seattle, WA: University of Washington, Seattle Press. (PMID 20301628).

[51] *Gale Encyclopedia of Genetic Disorders.* 2002. "Crouzon syndrome." Accessed December 24, 2018. https://www.encyclopedia.com/ science/ encyclopedias-almanacs-transcripts-and-maps/ crouzon-syndrome

[52] Ibrahimi, O.A., Chiu, E.S., McCarthy, J.G., and Mohammadi, M. 2005. "Understanding the molecular basis of Apert syndrome." *Plast Reconstr Surg* 115(1):264-270.

[53] Azaiez, H., Yang, T., Prasad, S., Sorensen, J.L., Nishimura, C.J., Kimberling, W.J., and Smith, R.J. 2007. "Genotype-phenotype correlations for SLC26A4- related deafness." *Hum Genet* 122, 451-457.

[54] Fraser, G.R. 1965. "Association of congenital deafness with goiter (Pendred's syndrome). A study of 207 families." *Ann Hum Genet* 28, 201-249.

[55] Illum, P., Kiaer, H.W., Hvidberg-Hansen, J., and Sondergaard, G. 1972. "Fifteen cases of Pendred's syndrome. Congenital deafness and sporadic goiter." *Arch Otolaryngol* 96, 297-304.

[56] Bizhanova, A., and Kopp, P. 2010. "Genetics and phenomics of Pendred syndrome." *Mol Cell Endocrinol* 322(1-2):83-90.

[57] Albert, S., Blons, H., Jonard, L., Feldman, D., Chauvin, P., Loundon, N., Sergent-Allaoui, A., Houang, M., Joannard, A., Schmerber, S., Delobel, B., Leman, J., Journel, H., Catros, H., Dollfus, H., Eliot, M.M., David, A., Calais, C., Drouin-Garraud, V., Obstoy, M.F., Tran Ba Huy, P., Lacombe, D., Duriez, F., Francannet, C., Bitoun, P., Petit, C., Garabedian, E.N., Couderc, R., Marlin, S., and Denoyelle, F. 2006. "SLC26A4 gene is frequently involved in nonsyndromic hearing impairment with enlarged vestibular aqueduct in Caucasian populations." *Eur J Hum Genet* 14, 773-779.

[58] Park, H.J., Shaukat, S., Liu, X.Z., Hahn, S.H., v, S., Ghosh, M., Kim, H.N., Moon, S.K., Abe, S., Tukamoto, K., Riazuddin, S., Kabra, M., Erdenetungalag, R., Radnaabazar, J., Khan, S., Pandya, A., Usami, S.I., Nance, W.E., Wilcox, E.R., and Griffith, A.J. 2003. "Origins and frequencies of SLC26A4 (PDS) mutations in east and south Asians: global implications for the epidemiology of deafness." *J Med Genet* 40, 242-248.

[59] Lentz, J., and Keats, B.J.B. 2016. "Usher syndrome type I." In *Gene Reviews*, edited by M.P. Adam, H.H. Ardinger, R.A. Pagon, Wallace, S.E., Bean, L.J.H., Stephens, K., and Amemiya, A. Seattle, WA: University of Washington, Seattle Press. (PMID 20301442).

[60] Umrigar, A., Musso, A., Mercer, D., Hurley, A., Glausier, C., Bakeer, M., Marble, M., Hicks, C., and Tsien, F. 2017. "Delayed

diagnosis of a patient with Usher syndrome 1C in a Louisiana Acadian family highlights the necessity of timely genetic testing for the diagnosis and management of congenital hearing loss." *SAGE Open Med Case Rep* 5:2050313X17745904.

[61] Gorlin, R.J. 1995. "Genetic hearing loss associated with eye disorders." In *Hereditary Hearing Loss and its Syndromes*, edited by R.J. Gorlin, H.V. Toriello, and M.M. Cohen. New York: Oxford University Press.

[62] Vernon, M. 1969. "Usher's syndrome- deafness and progressive blindness. Clinical cases, prevention, theory, and literature survey." *J Chronic Dis* 22:133-151.

[63] Yan, D., and Liu, X.Z. 2010. "Genetics and pathological mechanisms of Usher syndrome." *J Hum Genet* 55:327-335.

[64] Wahl, R.A., and Dick II, M. 1980. "Congenital deafness with cardiac arrhythmias: the Jervell and Lange-Nielsen syndrome." *Am Ann Deaf* 125, 34- 37.

[65] Kang, S.L., Jackson, C., and Kelsall, W. 2011. "Electrocardiogram screening of deaf children for long QT syndrome: are we following UK national guidelines?" *J Laryngol Otol* 125, 354-356.

[66] Tranebjaerg, L., Samson, R.A., and Green, G.E. 2017. "Jervell and Lange- Nielsen syndrome." In *Gene Reviews*, edited by M.P. Adam, H.H. Ardinger, R.A. Pagon, Wallace, S.E., Bean, L.J.H., Stephens, K., and Amemiya, A. Seattle, WA: University of Washington, Seattle Press. (PMID 20301579).

[67] Kruegel, J., Rubel, D., and Gross, O. 2013. "Alport syndrome- insights from basic and clinical research." *Nat Rev Nephrol* 10, 170-178.

[68] Pajari, H., Kaariainen, H., Muhonen, T., and Koskimies, O. 1996. "Alport's syndrome in 78 patients: epidemiological and clinical study." *Acta Paediatr* 85, 1300-1306.

[69] Alport Syndrome Foundation. 2017. *What is Alport Syndrome?* Accessed November 11, 2018. https://alportsyndrome.org/what-is-alport-syndrome/

[70] Kashtan, C.E. 2004. "Familial hematurias: what we know and what we don't." *Pediatr Nephrol* 20(8):1027-1035.

[71] Slajpah, M., Gorinsek, B., Berginc, G., Vizjak, A., Ferluga, D., Hvala, A., Meglic A., Jaksa, I., Furlan, P., Gregoric, A., Kaplan-Pavlovcic, S., Ravnik-Glavac, M., and Glavac, D. 2007. "Sixteen novel mutations identified in COL4A3, COL4A4, and COL4A5 genes in Slovenian families with Alport syndrome and benign familial hematuria." *Kidney Int* 71(12):1287-1295.

[72] Hertz, J.M., Thomassen, M., Storey, H., and Flinter, F. 2012. "Clinical utility gene card for: Alport syndrome." *Eur J Hum Genet* 20.

[73] Sproule, D.M., and Kaufmann, P. 2009. "Mitochondrial encephalopathy, lactic acidosis, and stroke-like episodes: basic concepts, clinical phenotype, and therapeutic management of MELAS syndrome." *Ann N Y Acad Sci* 1142:133-158.

[74] DiMauro, S. and Hirano, M. 2015. "MERRF." In *Gene Reviews*, edited by M.P. Adam, H.H. Ardinger, R.A. Pagon, Wallace, S.E., Bean, L.J.H., Stephens, K., and Amemiya, A. Seattle, WA: University of Washington, Seattle Press. (PMID 20301693).

[75] Sherman, S.L., Allen, E.G., Bean, L.H., and Freeman, S.B. 2007. "Epidemiology of Down syndrome." *Ment Retard Dev Disabil Res Rev* 13(3):221-227.

[76] National Center for Biotechnology Information. 2018. *Ensembl-Chromosome 21*. Accessed December 25, 2018. http://useast.ensembl.org/ Homo_sapiens/ Location/ Chromosome?chr=21; r=21:1-46709983

[77] Bull, M.J., and the Committee on Genetics. 2011. "Health supervision for children with Down syndrome." *Pediatrics* 128 :393-406.

[78] Nightengale, E., Yoon, P., Wolter-Warmerdam, K., Daniels, D., and Hickey, F. 2017. "Understanding hearing and hearing loss in children with Down syndrome." *Am J Audiol* 26(3):301-308.

[79] Hilgert, N., Smith, R.J.H., and Van Camp, G. 2009. "Forty-six genes causing nonsyndromic hearing impairment: which ones should be analyzed in DNA diagnostics?" *Mutat Res* 681, 189-196.

[80] Kenneson, A., Van Naarden Braun, K., and Boyle, C. 2002. "GJB2 (connexin 26) variants and nonsyndromic sensorineural hearing loss: a HuGE review." *Genet Med* 4, 258-274.

[81] Rabionet, R., Gasparini, P., and Estivill, X. 2000. "Molecular genetics of hearing impairment due to mutations in gap junction genes encoding beta connexins." *Hum Mutat* 16(3):190-202.

[82] Angeli, S., Lin, X., and Liu, X.Z. 2012. "Genetics of hearing and deafness." *Anat Rec* 295, 1812-1829.

[83] Snoeckx, R.L., Huygen, P.L., Feldmann, D., Marlin, S., Denoyelle, F., Waligora, J., Mueller-Malesinska, M., Pollak, A., Ploski, R., Murgia, A., Orzan, E., Castorina, P., Ambrosetti, U., Nowakowska-Szyrwinska, E., Bal, J., Wiszniewski, W., Janecke, A.R., Nekahm-Heis, D., Seeman, P., Bendova, O., Kenna, M.A., Frangulov, A., Rehm, H.L., Tekin, M., Incesulu, A., Dahl, H.H., du Sart, D., Jenkins, L., Lucas, D., Bitner-Glindzicz, M., Avraham, K.B., Brownstein, Z., del Castillo, I., Moreno, F., Blin, N., Pfister, M., Sziklai, I., Toth, T., Kelley, P.M., Cohn, E.S., Van Maldergem, L., Hilbert, P., Roux, A.F., Mondain, M., Hoefsloot, L.H., Cremers, C.W., Lopponen, T., Lopponen, H., Parving, A., Gronskov, K., Schrivjer, I., Roberson, J., Gualandi, F., Martini, A., Lina-Granade, G., Pallares-Ruiz, N., Correia, C., Fialho, G., Cryns, K., Hilgert, N., Van de Heyning, P., Nishimura, C.J., Smith, R.J., and Van Camp, G. 2005. "GJB2 mutations and degree of hearing loss: a multicenter study." *Am J Hum Genet* 77, 945-957.

[84] Mahdieh, N., and Rabbani, B. 2009. "Statistical study of 35delG mutation of GJB2 gene: a meta-analysis of carrier frequency." *Int J Audiol* 48, 363-370.

[85] Denoyelle, F., Martin, S., Weil, D., Moatti, L., Chauvin, P., Garabedian, E.N., and Petit, C. 1999. "Clinical features of the prevalent form of childhood deafness, DFNB1, due to a connexin-26

gene defect: implications for genetic counselling." *Lancet* 353, 1298-1303.

[86] Rehman, A.U., Bird, J.E., Faridi, R., Shahzad, M., Shah, S., Lee, K., Khan, S.N., Imtiaz, A., Ahmed, Z.M., Riazuddin, S., Santos-Cortez, R.L.P., Ahmad, W., Leal, S.M., Riazuddin, S., and Friedman, T.B. 2016. "Mutational spectrum of *MYO15A* and the molecular mechanisms of DFNB3 human deafness." *Hum Mutat* 37(10), 991-1003.

[87] Miyagawa, M., Nishio, S.Y., Hattori, M., Moteki, H., Kobayashi, Y., Sato, H., Watanabe, T., Naito, Y., Oshikawa, C., and Usami, S. 2015. "Mutations in the MYO15A gene are a significant cause of nonsyndromic hearing loss: massively parallel DNA sequencing-based analysis." *Ann Otol Rhinol Laryngol* 124 Suppl 1:158S-168S.

[88] Nal, N., Ahmed, Z.M., Erkal, E., Alper, O.M., Luleci, G., Dinc, O., Waryah, A.M., Ain, Q., Tasneem, S., Husnain, T., Chattaraj, P., Riazuddin, S., Boger, E., Ghosh, M., Kabra, M., Riazuddin, S., Morell, R.J., and Friedman, T.B. 2007. "Mutational spectrum of MYO15A: the large N-terminal extension of myosin XVA is required for hearing." *Hum Mutat* 28(10):1014-1019.

[89] Varga, R., Avenarius, M.R., Kelley, P.M., Keats, B.J., Berlin, C.I., Hood, L.J., Morlet, T.G., Brashears, S.M., Starr, A., Cohn, E.S., Smith, R.J.H., and Kimberling, W.J. 2006. "OTOF mutations revealed by genetic analysis of hearing loss families including a potential temperature sensitive auditory neuropathy allele." *J Med Genet* 43(7):576-581.

[90] Siemens, J., Kazmierczak, P., Reynolds, A., Sticker, M., Littlewood-Evans, A., and Muller, U. 2002. "The Usher syndrome proteins cadherin 23 and harmonin form a complex by means of PDZ-domain interactions." *PNAS* 99(23):14946-14951.

[91] Kazmierczak, P., Sakaguchi, H., Tokita, J., Wilson-Kubalek, E.M., Milligan, R.A., Muller, U., and Kachar, B. 2007. "Cadherin 23 and protocadherin 15 interact to form tip-link filaments in sensory hair cells." *Nature* 449:87-91.

[92] Schultz, J.M., Yang, Y., Caride, A.J., Filoteo, A.G., Penheiter, A.R., Lagziel, A., Morell, R.J., Mohiddin, S.A., Fananapazir, L., Madeo, A.C., Penniston, J.T., and Griffith, A.J. 2005. "Modification of human hearing loss by plasma- membrane calcium pump PMCA2." *New Eng J Med* 352:1557-1564.

[93] Kitajiri, S.I., McNamara, R., Makishima, T., Husnain, T., Zafar, A.U., Kittles, R.A., Ahmed, Z.M., Friedman, T.B., Riazuddin, S., and Griffith, A.J. 2007. "Identities, frequencies, and origins of TMC1 mutations causing DFNB7/B11 deafness in Pakistan." *Clin Genet* 72:546-550.

[94] Kurima, K., Peters, L.M., Yang, Y., Riazuddin, S., Ahmed, Z.M., Naz, S., Arnaud, D., Drury, S., Mo, J., Makishima, T., Ghosh, M., Menon, P.S., Deshmukh, D., Oddoux, C., Ostrer, H., Khan, S., Riazuddin, S., Deininger, P.L., Hampton, L.L., Sullivan, S.L., Battey, J.F., Jr., Keats, B.J., Wilcox, E.R., Friedman, T.B., and Griffith, A.J. 2002. "Dominant and recessive deafness caused by mutations of a novel gene, TMC1, required for cochlear hair-cell function." *Nat Genet* 30:277-284.

[95] Makishima, T., Kurima, K., Brewer, C.C., and Griffith, A.J. 2004. "Early onset and rapid progression of dominant nonsyndromic DFNA36 hearing loss." *Otol Neurotol* 25:714-719.

[96] Lee, Y.J., Park, D., Kim, S.Y., and Park, W.J. 2003. "Pathogenic mutations but not polymorphisms in congenital and childhood onset autosomal recessive deafness disrupt the proteolytic activity of TMPRSS3." *J Med Genet* 40(8):629-631.

[97] Weegerink, N.J., Schraders, M., Oostrik, J., Huygen, P.L., Strom, T.M., Granneman, S., Pennings, R.J., Venselaar, H., Hoefsloot, L.H., Elting, M., Cremers, C.W., Admiraal, R.J., Kremer, H., and Kunst, H.P. 2011. "Genotype-phenotype correlation in DFNB8/10 families with TMPRSS3 mutations." *J Assoc Res Otolaryngol* 12(6):753-766.

[98] Plantinga, R.F., de Brouwer, A.P., Huygen, P.L., Kunst, H.P., Kremer, H., and Cremers, C.W. 2006. "A novel TECTA mutation in a Dutch DFNA8/12 family confirms genotype-phenotype correlation." *J Assoc Res Otolaryngol* 7(2):173-181.

[99] Hughes, D.C., Legan, P.K., Steel, K.P., and Richardson, G.P. 1998. "Mapping of the alpha-tectorin gene (TECTA) to mouse chromosome 9 and human chromosome 11: a candidate for human autosomal dominant nonsyndromic deafness." *Genomics* 48(1):46-51.

[100] Minami, S.B., Masuda, S., Usui, S., Mutai, H., and Matsunaga, T. 2012. "Comorbidity of GJB2 and WFS1 mutations in one family." *Gene* 501(2): 193-197.

[101] Urano, F. 2016. "Wolfram syndrome: diagnosis, management, and treatment." *Curr Diab Rep* 16(1):6.

[102] Coucke, P., Van Camp, G., Djoyodiharjo, B., Smith, S.D., Frants, R.R., Padberg, G.W., Darby, J.K., Huizing, E.H., Cremers, C., Kimberling, W.J., Oostra, B.A., Van de Heyning, P.H., and Willems, P.J. 1994. "Linkage of autosomal dominant hearing loss to the short arm of chromosome 1 in two families." *N Engl J Med* 331:425-431.

[103] Van Camp, G., Coucke, P.J., Kunst, H., Schatteman, I., Van Velzen, D., Marres, H., van Ewijk, M., Declau, F., Van Hauwe, P., Meyers, J., Kenyon, J., Smith, S.D., Smith, R.J.H., Djelantik, B., Cremers, C.W.R.J., Van de Heyning, P.H., and Willems, P.J. 1997. "Linkage analysis of progressive hearing loss in five extended families maps the DFNA2 gene to a 1.25-Mb region on chromosome 1p." *Genomics* 41(1):70-74.

[104] Marres, H., van Ewijk, M., Huygen, P., Kunst, H., Van Camp, G., Coucke, P., Willems, P., and Cremers, C. 1997. "Inherited nonsyndromic hearing loss: an audiovestibular study in a large family with autosomal dominant progressive hearing loss related to DFNA2." *Arch Otolaryngol Head Neck Surg* 123:573-577.

[105] Jones, S.M., Robertson, N.G., Given, S., Giersch, A.B.S., Liberman, M.C., and Morton, C.C. 2011. "Hearing and vestibular deficits in the Coch(-/-) null mouse model: comparison to the Coch(G88E/G88E) mouse and to DFNA9 hearing and balance disorder." *Hear Res* 272(1-2):42-48.

[106] Fransen, E., Verstreken, M., Verhagen, W.I., Wuyts, F.L., Huygen, P.L., D'Haese, P., Robertson, N.G., Morton, C.C., McGuirt, W.T.,

Smith, R.J., Declau, F., Van de Heyning, P.H., and Van Camp, G. 1999. "High prevalence of symptoms of Meniere's disease in three families with a mutation in the COCH gene." *Hum Mol Genet* 8(8):1425-1429.

[107] Iossa, S., Marciano, E., and Franze A. 2011. "GJB2 gene mutations in syndromic skin diseases with sensorineural hearing loss." *Curr Genomics* 12, 475-485.

[108] Bademci, G., Lasisi, A.O., Yariz, K.O., Montenegro, P., Menendez, I., Vinueza, R., Paredes, R., Moreta, G., Subasioglu, A., Blanton, S., Fitoz, S., Incesulu, A., Sennaroglu, L., and Tekin, M. 2015. "Novel domain-specific POU3F4 mutations are associated with X-linked deafness: examples from different populations." *BMC Med Genet* 16:9. Accessed December 23, 2018. doi:10.1186/s12881-015-0149-2.

[109] de Melo, C.E.F.S., Ferreira, T.C., Higino, T.C.M., Maia, M.S., and Boccalini, M.C.C. 2010. "Gusher in stapedotomy- a case report." *Int Arch Otolaryngol* 14(2). Accessed November 23, 2018. doi:10.7162/S1809- 48722010000200015.

[110] Li, Z., Li, R., Chen, J., Liao, Z., Zhu, Y., Qian, Y., Xiong, S., Heman-Ackah, S., Wu, J., Choo, D.I., and Guan, M.X. 2005. "Mutational analysis of the mitochondrial 12S rRNA gene in Chinese pediatric subjects with amino- glycoside-induced and non-syndromic hearing loss." *Hum Genet* 117(1): 9-15.

[111] Bindu, L.H., and Reddy, P.P. 2008. "Genetics of aminoglycoside-induced and prelingual non-syndromic mitochondrial hearing impairment: a review." *Int J Audiol* 47(11):702-707.

[112] Qian, Y., and Guan, M.X. 2009. "Interaction of aminoglycosides with human mitochondrial 12S rRNA carrying the deafness-associated mutation." *Antimicrob Agents Chemother* 53(11):4612-4618.

[113] Prezant, T.R., Agapian, J.V., Bohlman, M.C., Bu. X., Oztas, S., Qiu, W.Q., Arnos, K.S., Cortopassi, G.A., Jaber, L., and Rotter, J.I. 1993. "Mito- chondrial ribosomal RNA mutation associated with both

antibiotic-induced and non-syndromic deafness." *Nat Genet* 4(3):289-294.

[114] Howe, B., Umrigar, A., and Tsien, F. 2014. "Chromosome preparation from cultured cells." *J Vis Exp* 83:e50203. Accessed December 22, 2018. doi: 10.3791/50203.

[115] Joint Committee on Infant Hearing. 2007. "Year 2007 position statement: principles and guidelines for early hearing detection and intervention programs." *Pediatrics* 120(4):898-921.

[116] Mercer, D. 2015. "Guidelines for audiologists on the benefits and limitations of genetic testing." *Am J Audiol* 24(4):451-461.

[117] Fowler, K.B., McCollister, F.P., Sabo, D.L., Shoup, A.G., Owen, K.E., Woodruff, J.L., Cox, E., Mohamed, L.S., Choo, D.I., and Boppana, S.B. 2017. "A targeted approach for congenital cytomegalovirus screening within newborn hearing screening." *Pediatrics* 139(2). Accessed December 24, 2018. doi:10.1542/peds.2016-2128.

[118] *National Society of Genetic Counselors*. 2018. Accessed December 26, 2018. https://www.nsgc.org.

In: Advances in Audiology Research
Editor: Victor M. Kristensen
ISBN: 978-1-53615-260-9
© 2019 Nova Science Publishers, Inc.

Chapter 2

AUDIOLOGICAL AND SURGICAL OUTCOME AFTER COCHLEAR IMPLANT REVISION SURGERY

Mohamed Salah Elgandy[1,2,*], *Marlan R. Hansen*[2,3]
and Richard S. Tyler[2,4]

[1]Department of Otolaryngology-Head and Neck Surgery,
Zagazig University, Egypt
[2]Department of Otolaryngology-Head and Neck Surgery,
University of Iowa, Iowa City, IA, US
[3]Department of Neurosurgery,
University of Iowa, Iowa City, IA, US
[4]Department of Communication Sciences and Disorders,
University of Iowa, Iowa City, IA, US

---

[*] Corresponding Author's E-mail: drmoh-ent@yahoo.com.

Abstract

Cochlear implantation is now widely accepted as a safe and effective treatment for children and adults with profound deafness. As with all electronic devices, a cochlear implant (CI) is susceptible to breakdown or failure. Although the CI reliability rate is now very high, the continually increasing population of implant recipients will result in the continued need for revision surgeries. The first report of a CI revision surgery occurred in 1985, by Hochmair-Desoyer and Burian. Since then, several reports have addressed the safety of this procedure, including the preservation or increase of speech per ception performance, although there have also been reports of decreases in electrode activation, decreased speech per ception and intra cochlear trauma, suggesting that cochlear reimplantation may have negative functional consequences in some patients, requiring careful consideration of the expected indications and benefits. This paper will review causes of revision surgery, how to diagnose cases of failed CI and will discuss surgical and audiological outcome of revision CI surgeries, Speech recognition ability with a replacement CI may significantly increase or decrease from that with the original implant. Experienced CI patients facing reimplantation must be counseled regarding the possibility of differences in sound quality and speech recognition performance with their replacement device.

Keywords: cochlear implant failure, revision surgery, surgical outcome, auditory performance

Introduction

Cochlear implant (CI) surgery began over 30 years ago. During the subsequent decades, auditory performance has improved, resulting in broader implantation criteria. As the number of implanted patients grows and the lifespan of devices is outlived, an increasing number of device failures are expected. In consequence, the odds of ensuing complications are higher. Therefore, analyzing performance and complications after revision cochlear implantation is of the utmost importance [1].

Revision surgery has always been cause for concern because of the potential risk of creating greater damage to delicate inner ear structures when removing the original device and replacing it with a new one.

Moreover, there is the fear of not being able to follow the path of the original electrode and achieve the same depth of insertion. Lastly, there is the possibility that functional performance will not be restored to levels achieved prior to device failure. This is of particular concern for the pediatric population in view of the fact that most children with CIs are pre linguistically deafened and are in the process of developing spoken communication skills. Disruption of sound input in the short term coupled with potential decrements in performance are serious consequences for the child requiring revision implant surgery. Owing to these potential adverse effects, investigating the prevalence of revision surgery and performance outcomes remains essential to clinical practice [2].

CAUSES OF REIMPLANTATION

Causes for reimplantation follow the classification proposed by Zeitler [3]. They include hard failure, soft failure, device infection or extrusion, improper initial placement, wound or flap complications, and upgrade of cochlear implant technology.

Device Failure

Hard failure occurs when there no auditory stimulation resulting from a confirmed malfunction of a component of the cochlear implant device; this might result from head trauma especially in children preventing communication between the internal and external components. Hard failures may be heralded by a sudden failure or an abnormal sound and no link to the processor. It is diagnosed by failed integrity test [3].

Soft failures are typically more challenging to recognize because the recipient has improved hearing compared to preimplantation and many factors are known to affect growth of auditory skills. Among all CI recipients, improvements in speech perception and localization varies widely across individuals Tyler et al. [4].

Table 1. Check list symptoms for soft failure in both young children and adults

Young children	
A- behavioral	• Increase in bad behavior • Aggressiveness • Un willing to wear device • Inattentiveness • Regression in speech/language
B-teacher\therapist concern	• Intermittent responsiveness • Frequent appearance of being off task • Deterioration of school performance • Plateau in performance • Failure to meet appropriate expectations
C- other factors	• Educational placement • Type and amount of therapy • Familial involvement • Puberty
Older children/adults	
A-auditory	• atypical tinnitus • buzzing • roaring • engine like noise • static • popping
B-non auditory	• pain over implant site • pain down neck • shocking • itching • fascial stimulations
C-performance	• sudden drop in performance • decrement in performance over time • failure to meet expected performance • intermittent performance
D- mapping	• change in levels over time • changes in pulse width\duration • loss of channels • type and amount of therapy • change in impedance • shorts/open circuits
E-hard ware	• replacements of all externals
F-objective assessment	• surface potential testing • neural response measures • evoked potentials • stimulus artifact

Symptoms of soft failure can be subtle and include decreased performance and speech perception, poor performance relative to expectations based on preimplantation characteristics, aversive stimuli causing subjective discomfort or pain especially at low stimulation levels, and hearing static while the device is off.

A frequent need for reprogramming or difficulty programming often mis-attributed to complicated patients may be related to the device. A strong index of suspicion may be needed to detect accompanying signs [5].

Balkany TJ et al. [6] suggested a checklist to evaluate soft failure in both children and adults.

Scalp Infection

Device infection may appear in the form of redness and fluctuation of the skin located over the receiver stimulator or an ulcerated wound. Once an infection or exposure of the device is suspected, antibiotics should be initiated immediately. If the infection persists, the explantation of the device is recommended.

According to Cohen [7], minor scalp flap complications are those that require minimal treatment or no treatment. They are less frequently reported than major complications. Signs of flap infection should be immediately recognized and treated. Local symptoms and signs include erythema, warmth, and drainage and crusting at the incision site.

Major scalp complications, include flap necrosis is often the result of poorly planned/executed incisions or flap designs. In patients with previous post auricular or face-lift incisions consideration should be given to modifications of the standard anteriorly based, C-shaped flap, as the blood supply to the flap may be inadequate. A "lazy S," straight, or inverted U- or J-flap have been proposed to improve survival of the flap. Infection and/or underlying inflammatory conditions (e.g., vasculitis) may also predispose to flap necrosis and problems with wound healing. There have been case reports acclaiming the use of hyperbaric oxygen to speed recovery/healing and even to "prepare" the bed for rotational flap.

Electrode Extrusion

Extra cochlear electrode extrusion is also an indication for revision surgery and may be suggested by a decline in speech perception for which there is no alternative explanation. After device-related indications, it is the most common cause of need for re implantation in children [8].

The exact etiology is unknown, but it may be related to initial misplacement, cochlear ossification, aggressive host inflammatory responses to the implanted biomaterials, or physical forces placed on the cochlea that pull the electrode out of position. This latter circumstance might manifest with a progressive decline in performance over time. Despite the intuitiveness of this theory as it relates to skull growth in patients implanted when they were young children, studies have not documented electrode migration in the developing pediatric population. The slow decline in speech perception found in these patients before revision CI suggests that extrusion may be a dynamic process that can progress.

Some theorize that the use of perimodiolar electrodes which are stable by hugging the modiolus may decrease the likelihood of electrode extrusion. Additionally, tightly packing the cochleostomy site may aid in keeping the electrode in place [9].

Cochlear Implant Electrode Misplacement

The standard location for insertion of the CI electrode array is into the scala tympani of the cochlea. Failure to insert the electrode array into the scala tympani has been documented in the literature [10]. This can range from misplacement of the electrode array into the vestibule or internal auditory canal, placement into scala vestibuli or scala media or, more commonly, translocation of an array that is initially placed in scala tympani into the scala media or vestibuli as the electrode array advances apically. Fortunately, misplacement of the electrode array into extra cochlear locations (e.g., vestibule) considered to be a major complication is rare.

Inner ear malformations increase the likelihood of electrode array misplacement. Preoperative radiographic examination should help to avoid such complications. Yet, a normal preoperative CT scan does not exclude inner ear malformation that could lead to misplacement of the electrode array, such as malformation of the osseous spiral lamina. In addition, incomplete ossification of the tympano meningeal fissure (Hyrtl's fissure) that usually occurs by the 24th week in utero can result in permanent patency and provide another potential route for extra cochlear misplacement of the electrode array.

Jain and Mukherji [11] reported that the electrode array may be misplaced into the middle ear cavity, mastoid bowl, cochlear aqueduct, petrous carotid canal, Eustachian tube, or may be only partially inserted into the cochlea. The electrode may also be inserted into the vestibular system, most commonly the superior or lateral semicircular canal. Therefore, vestibular symptoms that are associated with cochlear implantation should arouse suspicion of electrode array misplacement. In addition, electrode array malposition should be considered in all cases when no benefit is achieved, and should be evaluated both by device-integrity testing and CT imaging, even in the setting of late presentation weeks after implant surgery.

Beyond extra cochlear misplacement; electrode array misplacement within the cochlea can also reduce overall performance. since clinical functional outcome would be expected to be quite different. Regarding mal insertion of cochlear electrode within the cochlea, various patterns have been recognized [12].

1. Tip Rollover. Some newer, peri modilar electrode arrays are particularly prone to a tip roll-over and in these cases intraoperative imaging is helpful to confirm appropriate placement [13].
2. Over insertion of array: placing it deeper into the cochlea than desired, resulting in absence of electrodes in the proximal basal turn of the cochlea where high-frequency information is typically delivered.

3. Atwist in the electrode, the electrode bends or twists over on itself.
4. partial electrode insertion, electrode not inserted completely.
5. Translocation of the electrode array into scala media or vestibuli: This complication is relatively common, especially for electrode arrays placed deep in the cochlear apex. It is associated with increased scarring/fibrosis, neural degeneration, and diminished performance [14].

Magnet Displacement

A potentially problematic complication after cochlear implantation is the migration or displacement of the internal magnet. For older implant models in which there was a ceramic case that houses the internal receiver, this is not an issue. The advantage of having a removable magnet stems largely from the possibility of obtaining postoperative magnetic resonance imaging (MRI) scans. In a simple outpatient procedure, the internal magnet can be removed, scan obtained, and the magnet replaced. As compared with MRI-compatible implants without a removable magnet, the quality of an MRI of the head in a patient with an implant with the magnet removed is far superior [15]. To facilitate MRIs, most newer model implants contain removable magnets; however, it is possible that these removable magnets are more prone to dislodgement.

In the most common scenario, a child sustains some trauma to the skull overlying the receiver, thereby causing the magnet to literally pop out of its bed within the housing. Children are likely at greater risk for this than adults as a result of their developing motor skills and associated play activities and thinner scalps. In such a scenario, the patient may notice a lack of function of the implant or a hard lump just underneath the skin adjacent to the scalp.

When a displaced magnet is encountered, the patient or family should be counseled to not wear the device until the magnet can be replaced as a result of the risk for injuring the skin flap. Fortunately the repair of the problem is relatively straightforward. In rare cases, if the magnet becomes dislodged on multiple occasions and there is a tear in the Silastic ring holding the magnet in place, the entire implant may have to be replaced [16].

SURGICAL STEPS

After detection of a problem with the CI device, all efforts will be made to reimplant within the shortest time feasible. The surgery should ideally be performed by an experienced CI team.

In cases in which anatomy is preserved, re implantation is typically surgery performed following the same surgical steps. After skin incision and elevation of the skin flap, dissection should be done meticulous to try and preserve the physical integrity of the electrode array, which is encapsulated in a fibrous sheath. The lead is followed to the facial recess, round window and cochleostomy site; if present, are identified. If the implant is being removed and the reimplantation is being staged for a later date (e.g., in cases of infection), the array lead is cut as close as possible near to the posterior tympanotomy. This enables removal of the implant body and proximal electrode lead, without tension on the intra cochlear array and the risk of either inadvertent electrode removal or trauma to the cochlea. In such staged cases, the intra cochlear electrode lead is left in situ as a stent to preserve a tract for subsequent implantation.

If the cochlea is to be reimplanted with a new device at the same time (e.g., a device failure), the area around the cochleostomy is prepared in advance of the array change. Generally the implanted array can gently be withdrawn from the cochlea under microscopic visualization. If necessary, an incision can be made into the fibrous sheath that had formed around the old electrode array. The new device is positioned the pocket under the scalp [17] and the new array is inserted carefully without disruption of the fibrous sheath. It is important to note that ideally the diameter of the new electrode array should be the same diameter or smaller than the original one. Rarely, there may be intra cochlear ossification or fibrosis that obscures the electrode tract. If so, this is often encountered around the cochleostomy and can be removed with micro rasps, picks or even a small diamond burr.

After the old array was removed, it was used for biofilm research [18], while the body and the attached lead were sent back to the manufacturer for cause-of-failure testing. If reimplantation is not planned at the same procedure, we left the electrode in the cochlea as a stent to prevent cochlear ossification and to facilitate reimplantation in the future.

Regarding insertion depth, reinsertion is usually a smooth step and results in a full insertion of the electrode array, but partial reinsertion may occur [19, 20]. Use an electrode array that is smaller or equal diameter of original one may help mitigate the risk of partial insertion.

If resistance to insertion is high, it would be wise to use straight electrode or styled array because these are stiffer and may over resistance when it is encountered.

The implant team should develop a surgical contingency plan if reinsertion is not possible. For example, intervening ossification and/or intra cochlear granulation tissue may prohibit reinsertion of the new electrode. The surgeon should not first propose the question, "Can we implant the other ear?" in the operating room. Rather, the implant team should evaluate the suitability of the contralateral ear before revision surgery and counsel the patient accordingly. In cases of soft failure not associated with adverse stimuli, implantation of the contralateral ear may obviate removal of a functional device.

SURGICAL OUTCOME

Insertion of an electrode into the scala tympani often causes trauma to the spiral ligament and basilar membrane in the area of the basal turn [21]. Many histologic studies have indicated that while cochlear explantation followed by reimplantation can result in additional cochlear trauma in some cases, the trauma does not preclude successful use of the device [22].

Insertion of an electrode into the scala tympani often causes trauma to the spiral ligament and basilar membrane in the area of the basal turn [23].

However, surgical trauma to an already damaged cochlea does not appear to affect neural stimulation or auditory performance with an implant [24, 25]. Mounting evidence suggests that stimulation of remaining neural elements occurs at the level of the spiral ganglion cells or higher up the auditory pathway, because some patients with no hair cells or dendrites and markedly reduced spiral ganglion cell counts have received substantial benefit from their cochlear implants.

Greenberg et al. [26] reported in guinea pig that there was no significant difference in pathology of single implanted or reimplanted cochleae.

Jackler et al. [27] reported that cochlear explanation followed by immediate reimplantation may be not accompanied by damage to cochlea or its neural population. However, in cases with marked granulation tissue proliferation at round window and scala tympani, incidence of trauma is high.

Shepherd et al. [28] reported the histopathologic change after cochlear reimplantation using long multichannel intra cochlear electrodes in the macaque, where electrode insertion trauma involving the osseous spiral lamina or basilar membrane was greater in the reimplanted cochleae and also resulted in more extensive loss of basal ganglion cells, particularly when proliferation of granulation tissue at the cochleostomy was identified.

Linthicum et al. [29] reported that reimplantation histopathology showed marked new bone formation fibrous tissue and low count of spiral ganglion cells compared to single implanted cochlea.

Fayad et al. [30] reported that new bone formation around electrode especially greatest in scala tympani of basal turn and spiral ganglion cell count was marked reduced c representing less than 10% of normal spiral ganglion cells.

Li et al. [31] by using a scoring system for damage to the lateral cochlear wall and a three-dimensional reconstruction method reported that marked level of new bone and fibrous tissue formation with cochlear re implantation. In addition they reported that insertional trauma to lateral cochlear wall play an important role in subsequent fibrosis and neo ossification following implantation and reimplantation. They also reported high levels of osteoprotegerin within the spiral ligament which may serve to inhibit bone remodeling and exposure of the underlying endosteum which may provide a nidus for inflammatory process to enhance ossification and inflammatory mediators may contribute to general increase in new bone formation.

The complications of cochlear reimplantation surgery can be summarized as follows:

1. Incomplete Electrode Extraction During Cochlear Implant Revision; Although the majority of revision operations are completed without complication, the current report demonstrates that one cannot universally assume that complete extraction of an indwelling cochlear implant electrode array will be straightforward. Kang et al. [32] reported 3 cases in which incomplete electrode removal with fracture of distal part of it inside cochlea and authors attributed that due to dense fibrous and bony tissue response at the cochleostomy site that extended into the cochlea. It is possible that, in some pediatric patients, a robust inflammatory response results in a fibrous and/or bony sheath that completely encases the array and fixes it within the cochlea, additionally, some patients had cochlear implants with intra cochlear positioners, which are designed to achieve juxtamodiolar positioning by displacing the array against the medial wall of the cochlea. It is possible that the shim like effect of the positioners contributed to the difficulties encountered during extraction of the electrode.
2. C.S.F leakage; was considered the the sole complication encountered during revision surgery in the past as reviewed by Lassig et al. [33] who reported 1 intraoperative outflow of CSF as the only surgical complication in 61 revision operations. Similarly, Buchman et al. [34] reported 1 instance of CSF leakage in 33 revision operations. Fayad et al. [35] also reported 2 occurrences of CSF leakage in 43 revision operations. Excessive cerebrospinal fluid (CSF) can access the cochlea through patent developmental

pathways of the otic capsule or after traumatic disruption of the temporal bone.
3. facial nerve injury; Facial nerve injury risk is also high in revision and re-implantation surgery. Presence of fibrosis in the mastoid bowl, which requires meticulous dissection with careful avoidance of the facial nerve to free the original electrode array. Adequate irrigation in order to prevent thermal injury is also important. The surgeon should be cautious about atypical positioning of the facial nerve in labyrinth abnormality cases [36].
4. Injury of the annulus or bony external auditory canal skin; due to marked thinning of canal in revision cases to identify anatomical landmarks will lead to cholesteatoma if it is not adequately repaired, retraction pockets and lastly protrusion of electrode through external auditory canal [37].
5. Perilymphatic fistula; through a cochleostomy and insertion trauma to the labyrinth may lead to postoperative vestibular problems. In addition, a serous labyrinthitis caused by electrode placement in the cochlea was suspected as being the possible etiology for vertigo in CI patients [38].
6. Acute mastoiditis, post traumatic wound breakdown and receiver-stimulator/magnet displacement occurred also as complications of revision surgery which are similar to primary surgery [39].

AUDIOLOGICAL OUTCOME

Cochlear implantation has been proven to be very effective surgery in rehabilitation of prelingual deaf children and post lingual deaf adult, but for some reasons, removal of cochlear implant may be required. For both child and family, it is a stressful condition as patient will undergo repeated surgery, a period of nonuse, and a period of rehabilitation again. There is also a greater concern about complications such as reduced performance following repeated surgery.

Here we will discuss audiological performance following revision cochlear implant surgery starting by impedance.

Although reimplantation is an undesirable consequence of cochlear implantation, many studies have shown good post-reimplantation results in terms of speech-perception scores [40, 41]. Only a few studies have reported patients who did not achieve the same perception scores after reimplantation [42].

In most, if not all, published studies, the period between first implantation, occurrence of the defect, and subsequent reimplantation was fairly long. For that reason, in most cases, a newer type of implant or another brand had become available and was implanted instead of the device that was initially used [43]. As a result, the newer device was an upgraded version of the former device and was coupled with improved software to drive the new implant. Hence, those changes in design, brand, or software could be the explanation of the same, or even better, speech-perception scores. Consequently, the confounding variable of a different type of implant weakens the comparison between speech- perception outcomes from the first implantation and the reimplantation.

Impedance

Impedance is a measure of electrical resistance at the electrode. it depends upon design of electrode, including materials used, surrounding tissues, fluid through which current exist and the electrode location into cochlea [44].

It can be increased by amount of cell cover and fibrous tissue growth around electrode array. As a result of repeated surgery there is increase in scar tissue formation and new bone and ossification. Thus increased impedance can be used post-operative as marker or proxy for increased inflammation [45]. High impedance is of clinical concern because it can cause saturation (compliance) of electrodes and reduce the dynamic range of stimulation.

Reduction in electrical impedance of cochlear implant electrodes is important as less energy is used, and this prolongs the cochlear battery life. Lower impedance with lower current allows for more focused stimulation of the neural elements in the cochlea, giving greater differentiation of sounds [46].

Neuburger et al. [47] found that increases in impedance are often accompanied by clinical inflammatory precipitation, with exudate and labyrinthitis and this can be in some cases of revision not all cases due to new bone formation with accompanying fibrosis.

Measurement of impedance will be conducted at time of surgery to identify very high impedance(open circuit) which is indicative of break in the wire lead, damage of electrode contact point, air bubbles around electrode contact, electrode malposition either (incomplete insertion or delayed extrusion) and ossification of cochlea fibrosis and inflammation, or low impedance (short circuit) which is indicator of one or two electrodes share a common electrical course, or partial short circuit which means that impedance decreased over time but failed to reach a value that will be flagged by software as a short circuit [48].

Steroids can decrease impedance levels and are used in hearing preservation techniques and cases with cochlear explant and reimplant which result in impedance elevation, although the duration of protection, areas of cochlea protected, and the best mode of delivery is still under investigation [49].

Speech Recognition

Does cochlear reimplantation affect speech recognition?

As electronic devices, cochlear implants are occasionally subject to damage or breakdowns. Obviously, in the event that a cochlear implant becomes unusable, reimplantation becomes necessary. Doubts may arise in the patient about his subsequent speech recognition performance with a new implant.

Hamzavi et al. [50] recently demonstrated substantial benefits in patients in whom an analogue single-channel implant was upgraded to a digital multichannel device. In that study, he observed that, 3 months following reimplantation, five of seven patients achieved speech recognition performance at about the same level experienced with the original implant. A decrease in speech recognition was noted in one subject only, and was related to her central auditory system.

Henson et al. [51] evaluated a group of 28 patients (Nucleus 22 cochlear implant) who were reimplanted. 37% of patients achieved significantly higher sentence or word scores with their replacement cochlear implants than with their original implants, while 26% showed no significant change. The reason for the decline in speech recognition in that group was unclear, and parameters such as insertion depth or surgical complications did not seem to be relevant.

Parisier et al. [52] analyzed the outcomes of cochlear reimplantation in 25 children provided with Nucleus 22 cochlear implants. They found that open-set speech recognition scores and speech perception abilities remained stable or improved compared with results before reimplantation.

Balkany et al. [53] also found the speech recognition scores following reimplantation to be at least as good as with their initial implant. To achieve further beneficial audiological performance upon reimplantation, it appears that the same conditions which were applied to the initial implantation, such as insertion depth, implant type, and number of active channels, might be important indicators, as described by Miyamoto et al. [54].

Manrique et al. [55] reported a study on 38 patients requiring reimplantation and found that aided pure-tone hearing thresholds improved in 44% of the reimplanted patients, with 11% showing no change in their threshold. 64% percent of the patients showed an improvement between 20% and 35% points in their disyllabic word recognition score after reimplantation, with a further 9% showing no change in their speech recognition scores (SRS) from before to after reimplantation.

Rivas et al. [56] reviewed 34 patients who underwent cochlear reimplant, scores after reimplantation were better in 65% of cases, the same in 32%, and worse in 3%, when compared with the score obtained just prior to reimplantation.

Mahtani et al. [57] reported 32 reimplantation surgeries for 30 patients and reported that For the 25 adults with available scores in the quiet condition, 56% had no change in scores after reimplantation, 36% had improved scores, and 8% had poorer scores. For the 16 recipients tested in noise, 50% demonstrated no significant difference after reimplantation, 25% obtained significantly better scores, and the 25% obtained significantly worse scores.

CONCLUSION

Although cochlear implant surgery has been proven as a safe and effective method in rehabilitation of postlingual deaf adult and prelingual deaf children, these devices are subjected to damage, breakdown, need to upgrade and failure. In such cases, reimplantation is necessary. Although surgical problems leading to revision surgery and reimplantation are expected to diminish by experience, every center has to deal with device failures. Both revision surgery and reimplantation require extra care and it should be better carried out by experienced surgeons. Implant performances are expected to be comparable with primary implantations and a lot of studies showed improve audiological outcome after reimplantation.

REFERENCES

[1] Lassig, AA; Zwolan, TA; Telian, SA. Cochlear implant failures and revision. *Otol Neurotol*, 2005, 26, 624–34.

[2] Weise, JB; Muller-Deile, J; Brademann, G; et al. Impact to the head increases cochlear implant reimplantation rate in children. *Auris Nasus Larynx*, 2005, 32, 39–43.

[3] Zeitler, DM; Budenz, CL; Roland, JL. Jr. (2009). Revision cochlear implantation. *Curr Opin Otolaryngol Head Neck Surg*, 17, 334–338.

[4] Tyler, RS; Parkinson, AJ; Woodworth, GG; Lowder, MW; Gantz, BJ. Performance over time of adult patients using the Ineraid and Nucleus cochlear implants. *Journal of the Acoustical Society of America*, (1997), 102(1), 508-522.

[5] Balkany, TJ; et al. Cochlear reimplantation. *Laryngoscope*, 1999, 109, 351–355.

[6] Balkany, TJ; et al. Cochlear implant soft failures consensus development conference statement. *Otol Neurotol*, 2005, 26, 815–818.

[7] Cohen, NL; Hoffman, RA; Stroschein, M. Medical or surgical complications related to the nucleus multichannel cochlear implant. *Ann Otol Rhinol Laryngol*, 135, 8-13, 1988.

[8] Brown, KD; Connell, SS; Balkany, TJ; Eshraghi, AE; Telischi, FF; Angeli, SA. Incidence and indications for revision cochlear implant surgery in adults and children. *Laryngoscope*, 2009, 119(1), 152–157.

[9] Ambyraja, R; Gutman, MA; Megrian, CA. Cochlear implant complications. *Arch Oto-Head Neck Surg*, 2005, 131, 245–250.

[10] Marlowe, Al; Chinnici, JE; Rivas, A; et al. Revision cochlear implant surgery in children: The Johns Hopkins experience. *Otol Neurotol*, 2010, 31, 74–82.

[11] Jain, R; Mukherji, SK. Cochlear implant failure: imaging evaluation of the electrode course. *Clin Radiol*, 2003, 58, 288–93.

[12] Hughes, M. *Objective measures in cochlear implants*. San Diego, CA: Plural Publishing, 2013.

[13] Zuniga, M. Geraldine; Rivas, Alejandro; Hedley-Williams, Andrea; Gifford, Rene H; Dwyer, Robert; Dawant, Benoit M; Sunderhaus, Linsey W; Hovis, Kristen L; Wanna, George B; Noble, Jack H; Labadie, Robert F. *Tip Fold-over in Cochlear Implantation Otology & Neurotology*, 38(2), February 2017, p. 199–206.

[14] Fischer, N; Pinggera, L; Weichbold, V; Dejaco, D; Schmutzhard, J; Widmann, G. Radiologic and Functional Evaluation of Electrode

Dislocation from the Scala Tympani to the Scala Vestibuli in Patients with Cochlear Implants. *American Journal of Neuroradiology*, February 2015, 36 (2), 372-377.

[15] 35-Migirov, L; Kronenberg, J. Magnet displacement following cochlear implantation. *Otol Neurotol*, 2005, 26, 646–648.

[16] 36-Yun, JM; Colburn, MW; Antonelli, PJ. Cochlear implant magnet displacement with minor head trauma. *Otolaryngol Head Neck Surg*, 2005, 133, 275–277.

[17] Lenarz, T. *Cochlea-implantat. Ein praktischer Leitfaden furs die Versorgung von Kindern und Erwachsenen.* [*Cochlear implant. A practical guide to the care of children and adults*]. Berlin: Springer, 1998

[18] Frijns-van Putten, A; Beers, M; Snieder, SG; Frijns, JHM. Hoortraining voor volwassen CI-dragers: Het cochleaire leer model [Hearing training for adult CI wearers: The cochlear leather model]. *Logopedie en Foniatrie*, 2005, 77, 50–59.

[19] Lassig, AA; Zwolan, TA; Telian, SA. Cochlear implant failures and revision. *Otol Neurotol*, 2005, 26, 624–634.

[20] Miyamoto, RT; Svirsky, MA; Myres, WA; Kirk, KI; Schulte, J. Cochlear implant reimplantation. *Am J Otol*, 1997, 18, S60–S61.

[21] Fayad, J; Linthicum, FH; Jr. Otto, SR; et al. Cochlear implants: histopathologic findings related to performance in 16 human temporal bones. *Ann Otol Rhinol Laryngol*, 1991, 100, 807-11.

[22] Miller, JM; Altschuler, RA; Carlisle, L; et al. Cochlear prosthesis: histologic observations on reimplantation in the monkey. In: *Abstracts of the Tenth Mid-Winter Research Meeting*. Clearwater Beach, FL: Association for Research in Otolaryngology, 1987, p. 54.

[23] Lehnhardt, M; Von Wallenberg, EL; Brinch, J. Cochlear implant reliability. *Fifth International Cochlear Implant Conference*, New York, NY, May 1-3, 1997.

[24] Hamzavi, J; Baumgartner, WD; Pok, SM. Does cochlear reimplantation affect speech recognition? *Int. J Audio*, 2002, 41, 151-6.

[25] Shepherd, RK; Graeme, MC; Xu, SA; et al. Cochlear pathology following reimplantation of a multi-channel scala tympani electrode array in the macaque. *Am J Otol*, 1995, 16, 186-99?

[26] Greenberg, AB; Myers, MW; Hartshorn, DO; Miller, JM; Altschuler, RA. Cochlear electrode reimplantation in the guinea pig. *Hear Res*, 1992, 61, 19–23.

[27] Jackler, RK; Leake, PA; McKerrow, WS. Cochlear implant revision: effects of reimplantation on the cochlea. *Ann Otol Rhinol Laryngol*, 1989, 98, 813–820.

[28] Shepherd, RK; Clark, GM; Xu, SA; Pyman, BC. Cochlear pathology following reimplantation of a multichannel scala tympani electrode array in the macaque. *Am J Otol*, 1995, 16, 186–199.

[29] Linthicum, FH; Jr. Fayad, J; Otto, SR; Galey, FR; House, WF. Cochlear implant histopathology. *Am J Otol*, 1991, 12, 245–311.

[30] Fayad, JN; Baino, T; Parisier, SC. Revision cochlear implant surgery: causes and outcome. *Otolaryngol Head Neck Surg*, 2004, 131, 429–432.

[31] Li, PMMC; Somdas, MA; Eddington, DK; Nadol, JB. Jr. Analysis of intra cochlear new bone and fibrous tissue formation in human subjects with cochlear implants. *Ann Otol Rhinol Laryngol*, 2007, 116, 731–738.

[32] Kang, SY; Zwolan, TA; Kileny, PR; Niparko, JK; Driscoll, CL; Shelton, C; Telian, SA. Incomplete electrode extraction during cochlear implant revision. *Otology and Neurotology*, 2009, 30(2), 160-164.

[33] Lassig, AA; Zwolan, TA; Telian, SA. Cochlear implant failures and revision. *Otol Neurotol*, 2005, 26, 624Y34.

[34] Buchman, CA; Higgins, CA; Cullen, R; et al. Revision cochlear implant surgery in adult patients with suspected device malfunction. *Otol Neurotol*, 2004, 25, 504Y10, discussion 10.

[35] Fayad, JN; Baino, T; Parisier, SC. Revision cochlear implant surgery: causes and outcome. *Otolaryngol Head Neck Surg*, 2004, 131, 429Y32.

[36] Kubo, K; Matsuura, S; Iwaki, T. Complications of cochlear implant surgery, *Oper. Tech. Otolaryngol.*, 16, (2005), 154–158.

[37] Lescanne, E; Zahrani, MA; Bakhos, D; Robier, A; Moriniere, S. Revision surgeries and medical interventions in young cochlear implant recipients, *Int. J. Pediatric. Otorhinolaryngol.*, 75, (2011), 1221–1224.

[38] Kubo, T; Yamamoto, K; Iwaki, T; Doi, K; Tamura, M. DiVerent forms of dizziness occurring after cochlear implant. *Eur Arch Otorhinolaryngol*, 2001, 258, 9–12.

[39] Kandogan, T; Olgun, L; Gu¨ntekin, G. Complications of paediatric cochlear implantations: experience in I˙ zmir, *J. Laryngol. Otol.*, 119 (8), (2005), 606–610.

[40] Alexiades, G; Roland, JT; Jr. Fishman, AJ; Shapiro, W; Waltzman, SB; Cohen, NL. Cochlear reimplantation: surgical techniques and functional results. *Laryngoscope*, 2001, 111, 1608–1613.

[41] Cote, M; Ferron, P; Bergeron, F; Bussieres, R. Cochlear reimplantation: causes of failure, outcomes, and audiologic performance. *Laryngoscope*, 2007, 117, 1225–1235.

[42] Henson, AM; Slattery, WH; III. Luxford, WM; Mills, DM. Cochlear implant performance after reimplantation: a multicenter study. *Am J Otol*, 1999, 20, 56–64.

[43] Lassig, AA; Zwolan, TA; Telian, SA. Cochlear implant failures and revision. *Otol Neurotol*, 2005, 26, 624–634.

[44] Paasche, G; Bockel, F; Tasche, C; Lesinski-Schiedat, A; Lenarz, T. Changes of postoperative impedances in cochlear implant patients: the short-term effects of modified electrode surfaces and intra cochlear corticosteroids. *Otol Neurotol*, 2006, 27, 639Y47.

[45] Newbold, C; Richardson, R; Huang, CQ; Milojevic, D; Cowan, R; Shepherd, R. An *in vitro* model for investigating impedance changes with cell growth and electrical stimulation: implications for cochlear implants. *J Neural Eng*, 2004, 1, 218Y27.

[46] Micco, AG; Richter, CP. Tissue resistivities determine the current flow in the cochlea. *Curr Opin Otolaryngol Head Neck Surg*, 2006, 14, 352Y5.

[47] Neuburger, J; Lenarz, T; Lesinski-Schiedat, A; Buchner, A. Spontaneous increases in impedance following cochlear implantation: suspected causes and management. *Int. J Audiol*, 2009, 48, 233Y9.

[48] Carlson, M; Archibald, D; Dabade, T; Gifford, R; Neff, B; Beatty, C; et al. Prevalence and timing of individual cochlear implant electrode failures. *Otol Neurotol.*, 2010, 31(6), 893–8.

[49] De Ceulaer, G; Johnson, S; Yperman, M; et al. Long-term evaluation of the effect of intra cochlear steroid deposition on electrode impedance in cochlear implant patients. *Otol Neurotol*, 2003, 24, 769Y74.

[50] Hamzavi, J; Baumgartner, WD; Adunka, O; Franz, P; Gstoettner, W. Audiological performances with cochlear reimplantation from analog single channel to digital multichannel devices. *Audiology*, (2000), 39, 305-10.

[51] Henson, AM; Slattery, WH; 3rd. Luxford, WM; Mills, DM. Cochlear implant performance after reimplantation: a multicenter study. *Am J Otol*, (1999), 20(1), 56-64.

[52] Parisier, SC; Chute, PM; Popp, AL; Suh, GD. Outcome analysis of cochlear implant reimplantation in children. *Laryngoscope*, (2001), 111(1), 26-32.

[53] Balkany, TJ; Hodges, AV; Gomez-Marin, O; et al. Cochlear reimplantation. *Laryngoscope*, (1999), 109(3), 351-5.

[54] Miyamoto, RT; Svirsky, MA; Myres, WA; Kirk, KI; Schulte, J. Cochlear implant reimplantation. *Am J Otol*, (1997), 18, 60-1.

[55] Manrique-Huarte, R; Huarte, A; Manrique, MJ. Surgical findings and auditory performance after cochlear implant revision surgery. *European Archives of Oto-Rhino-Laryngology*, (2016), 273(3), 621–629.

[56] Rivas, A; Marlowe, AL; Chinnici, JE; Niparko, JK; Francis, HW. Revision cochlear implantation surgery in adults: Indications and results. *Otology & Neurotology*, (2008), 29(5), 639–648.

[57] Mahtani, S; Glynn, F; Mawman, DJ; O'Driscoll, MP; Green, K; Bruce, I; Lloyd, SKW. Outcomes of cochlear reimplantation in adults. *Otology & Neurotology*, (2014), 35(8), 1366–1372.

In: Advances in Audiology Research
Editor: Victor M. Kristensen

ISBN: 978-1-53615-260-9
© 2019 Nova Science Publishers, Inc.

Chapter 3

THE RELATIONSHIP BETWEEN SELF-REPORTED RESTRICTION IN SOCIAL PARTICIPATION, SELF-REPORTED SATISFACTION/BENEFIT AND THE TIME OF USE OF HEARING AIDS

João Paulo N. A. Santos[1], Nathany L. Ruschel[2], Camila Z. Neves[3] and Adriane R. Teixeira[4],*

[1]Speech Therapy and Audiology Service,
Hospital de Clínicas de Porto Alegre, Porto Alegre,
Rio Grande do Sul, Brazil
[2]Child and Adolescent Health Post-Graduate Program,
Universidade Federal do Rio Grande do Sul, Porto Alegre,
Rio Grande do Sul, Brazil
[3]Comunicare Hearing Aids, Porto Alegre, Rio Grande do Sul, Brazil

---

* Corresponding Author's E-mail: adriane.teixeira@gmail.com.

[4]Health and Human Comunication Department, Universidade Federal do Rio Grande do Sul and Speech Therapy and Audiology Service, Hospital de Clínicas de Porto Alegre, Porto Alegre, Rio Grande do Sul, Brazil

Abstract

To correlate the results obtained through questionnaires concerning self-reported restriction in social participation and patient satisfaction/benefit with objective time assessment of device use. This is a descriptive, cross-sectional study sample composed of and elderly and non-elderly adults of both sexes diagnosed with hearing loss and approved as candidates for hearing aid fitting at a university hospital. Subjects answered questionnaires that measure restriction in social participation restriction and user satisfaction/benefit, namely the Hearing Handicap Inventory for Adults (HHIA) for non-elderly adult patients; the Hearing Handicap Inventory for the Elderly Screening Version (HHIE-S), for elderly patients, and the International Outcome Inventory for Hearing Aids (IOI-HA) for both age groups. Average daily usage time of the devices was verified objectively through datalogging. A total of 49 users elderly and non-elderly of both sexes participated in the study. Self-reported hearing aid times of use were compared with those measured by datalogging. There was overestimation on the part of patients when reporting hearing aid use, which was verified when compared with software data. There was no significant correlation between questionnaire scores and the datalogged time of use. There was a negative correlation between the HHIE-S and IOI-HA questionnaires, and a positive correlation between the variable of age and the IOI-HA questionnaire, as well as another positive correlation between the variable of sex and the HHIA questionnaire. No relation was found between datalogged time of use and self-reported restriction in social participation or hearing aid user satisfaction/benefit.

Keywords: hearing aids, hearing loss, questionnaires

Introduction

According to the National Health Survey of 2013, 1.1% of the Brazilian population - approximately 2.27 million people - are hearing impaired, with the South of the country representing the highest proportion of this indicator (1.5%). Research data also reveal that hearing loss is more frequent in the elderly (5.2%) or among people with lower levels of education or an incomplete elementary education. These findings are highly significant when compared to other data on age and education [1]. Hearing impairment causes disturbances in the social life of elderly patients as well as non-elderly adults and is also associated with other symptoms, such as depression, as well as functional and cognitive decline [2]. In relation to the elderly, it has been shown that hearing loss frequently entails a restriction in social participation and a lack of communicative competence; that is to say, it has a significant impact on the subjects' quality of life [3].

In the Brazilian Unified Health System (SUS), the cost-free fitting of hearing aids (HAs) has been granted since 2000. Public provision policies were amplified after the implementation of the Hearing Care Network for the Hearing Impaired and preceded the elaboration of the National Attention to Hearing Health policy. Since the implementation of these public protocols, demands for promotion, prevention and rehabilitation have been better met at federal, state and municipal levels [4, 5].

In order to facilitate a satisfactory hearing aid adaptation process, a speech-language pathologist qualified in audiology should carry out an appropriate HA selection and then give detailed and careful advice to the patient [6]. After fitting, successful adaptation also depends on the daily time of the use of the HA. This can be accurately measured through datalogging, a feature present in sound amplification devices. In order to validate success or setbacks in the adjustment process, the speech-language pathologist uses questionnaires to subjectively gauge patient satisfaction and benefit from hearing aid use [6]. In scientific literature, studies have been found that describe the importance of measuring user satisfaction/benefit in the process of adaptation. However, few studies correlate datalogged daily time of use with questionnaires that aim at validating the adaptation process.

It is known that the process of selecting and adapting to hearing aids aims to, among other goals, circumvent restrictions in social participation and help the user to effectively make use of their devices, thus favoring user satisfaction/benefit. In this sense, for a well-structured process of verification and validation, orientation, adaptation and self-assessment, questionnaires should be used in the best way possible [7].

Among the questionnaires used to evaluate patient hearing loss are the Hearing Handicap Inventory for Adults (HHIA) and the Hearing Handicap Inventory for the Elderly - Screening Version (HHIE-S) [8]. The first is used to verify participation restriction caused by hearing loss in non-elderly adults and the second is used to verify the same phenomenon in the elderly. Participation restriction or handicap is considered to be any disadvantage imposed by hearing impairment which limits an individual psychosocially. Many times elderly and non-elderly patients with hearing losses need to use hearing aids in order to compensate for the reported deficits caused by hypoacusia. Although these devices are used as a way to address negative social impacts, some accompanying strategies are even more decisive for their successful use, such as the elaboration of realistic expectations together with the patient regarding the compensation provided by the hearing aid. Moreover, appropriate advice and orientation by the speech-language pathologist directly supports patient adjustment, which in turn results in increased perception of satisfaction/benefit and a reduction in handicap [9].

Another necessary task for a speech and language pathologist who works with the selection and adaptation of HAs is to analyze self-reported user satisfaction and benefit. With this objective, after a minimal period of fifteen days post-fitting, the internationally used *Outcome Inventory for Hearing Aids* (IOI-HA) [10] can be applied to verify adjustment to the HA from the user's point of view. It takes into account daily evolution, degree of user satisfaction, impact on other people, restriction in social participation and limitations in basic activities. In addition, the IOI-HA questionnaire allows the patient to report the daily time of use of the hearing aid [11].

In peer-reviewed literature, there are few studies that correlate datalogging to the protocols mentioned previously, with the exception of the IOI-HA protocol. Some studies have found a significant correlation between the time of use of the hearing aid registered through datalogging and the self-reports of users, as well as a correlation between the time of use registered by datalogging with other protocols that measure patient satisfaction/benefit [12, 13]. Thus, the present study has as a general objective the correlation of findings regarding restrictions in social participation caused by the hearing loss, hearing aid user satisfaction/benefit and the datalogged times of use of these devices. Furthermore, our specific objectives are to analyze the relationship between the questionnaires themselves; to correlate the datalogged time of use and questionnaires with different variables such as age, education and type and degree of hearing loss. What is more, we aim to analyze the correlation between self-reported daily time of use and the datalogged time of use of these devices.

METHODS

The study was of the transversal and descriptive type. The sample consisted of elderly and non-elderly patients of both sexes who had been diagnosed with hearing loss by an Ear, Nose and Throat (ENT) specialist had gone through an audiological evaluation. These subjects were approved as candidates for hearing aid fitting and subsequently received these devices through the National Hearing Health Program at a university hospital.

Inclusion criteria were that recruited patients should sign an Informed Consent form (IC) and have undergone an ENT and audiological evaluation (pure tone audiometry, speech audiometry and acoustic impedance tests measures). Subjects who received their hearing aids via the program should have been using their devices for at least 15 days. Users under the age of 18 were excluded from the sample as well as patients who demonstrated partial or total incomprehension of the questionnaires due to cognitive, neurological or language issues.

In the process of selection and adaptation of the hearing aids, initial evaluations were carried out to verify the type and degree of hearing loss, along with the most appropriate type of device for each patient's needs. After fitting, patients received individual guidance on the proper use, handling and care of the devices. It should be noted that patients were not informed about the possibility of checking the time of use through datalogging.

After a minimal period of fifteen days, patients returned for a follow-up appointment. This period is a guideline at the outpatient clinic where the research was done. At that time, adjustments, verifications and further explanations about patients' hearing aids were performed, with the aim of guaranteeing continuity of use. Patients were also invited to participate in the research project. After signing the IC form, subjects were shown to a specific room in the outpatient clinic to answer questionnaires. At this stage, only the interviewer and the HA user were present in the interview room, in order to avoid interference from family members and caregivers.

First, subjects answered questionnaires regarding social participation restriction due to hearing loss: the HHIE-S questionnaire for elderly patients or the HHIA for non-elderly adult subjects. Next, the IOI-HA questionnaire was applied to assess user satisfaction/benefit. After, the datalogged daily time of use was verified for the subsequent analysis and correlation of the questionnaire scores and self-reported average daily time of use.

Questionnaires were applied during one-on-one interviews which were adjusted according to the level of education of each research participant. The differences between first two questionnaires, the HHIES-S and HHIA, lie in their distinct target populations as well as the overall number of questions. The former is a shorter version, containing ten questions, five of which address emotional aspects and the other five social/situational aspects. As such, the cut-off points that determine user participation are different than those of the HHIA, which is a questionnaire composed of twenty-five questions. As for the score, four points, two points and zero points were given for the answers "yes", "maybe" and "no", respectively. In both cases, the higher the score, the greater the self-reported restriction in social participation. The HHIE-S questionnaire has a total score of forty points: zero to eight points represents no perceived restriction in social participation, ten to twenty-three a mild to moderate restriction and twenty-four to forty a significant restriction. The HHIA questionnaire has a total score of 100 points: a score of zero to sixteen is indicative of no perceived restriction in social participation, eighteen to thirty points indicate slight restriction, thirty-two to forty points indicate moderate restriction and scores above forty-two points indicate a significant restriction in social participation [14].

The IOI-HA questionnaire was also applied during the interview. This particular instrument should be used within the first 15 days after hearing aid fitting. The questions take into account degree of user satisfaction/benefit, restrictions in social participation and limitations in basic activities [7]. It consists of seven questions, each worth a score of between one to five, where one represents the most negative response and five the most positive. The maximum score is thirty-five points, which is indicative of a very positive evaluation by the HA user, whereas the minimum score of five points is indicative of a negative evaluation by the HA user.

After the application of the questionnaires, an objective verification of time of use was carried out through the datalogging feature, which is present in all HAs distributed at the outpatient clinic. Data regarding sex, age and type and degree of hearing loss were also obtained through patients' electronic records.

The sample size calculation was performed in the WinPEPI program (*Programs for Epidemiologists for Windows*) version 11.43 [12, 13]. For a level of significance of 5%, to the power of 80%, and estimating a minimum correlation coefficient of 0.4 between the variables of satisfaction, benefit and restriction in social participation and time of use, a minimum total of 47 patients was obtained.

Quantitative variables were described by mean and standard deviation or interquartile range and median. Categorical variables were described by absolute and relative frequencies. To compare means between ears, the *t-student* test for paired samples was applied. In cases of asymmetry, the *Wilcoxon test* was used. For the categorical variables, the *McNemar* test was applied. To compare means between gender and type of loss, the *t-*

student test for independent samples or Analysis of Variance (ANOVA) were applied. In cases of asymmetry, the *Mann-Whitney* and *Kruskal-Wallis* tests were used. To evaluate the association between continuous and ordinal variables, the *Pearson* or *Spearman* correlation tests were applied. The significance level adopted was 5% ($p \leq 0.05$) and the analyses were performed though the SPSS program, version 21.0.

The present study was submitted to and approved by the Research Ethics Committee (CEP) of the institution, and approved (protocol number 2.086.280). Was regulated according to the norms concerning research involving human beings, duly governed by resolution 466/12 of the National Health Council.

Result

The present study consisted of a sample of 49 subjects, the majority of whom were elderly patients (71.42%). Among study subjects, there was equal distribution with regard to sex. Most of the participants in the sample had lower levels of education. The greater part of the group was fitted bilaterally with hearing aids (Table 1).

The HHIE-S questionnaire for the elderly presented a median of 6 and, for non-elderly adults, the HHIA median was 0. Thus, most of the study subjects, both elderly and non-elderly adults, declared no restriction in social participation after the use of HAs. The quantitative data collected through the IOI-HA questionnaire revealed an average score of 29.3 points, which is a good indication of HA user satisfaction/benefit (Table 1).

Regarding the type of hearing loss, the predominant profile was sensorineural, symmetrical, bilateral loss. The most frequent degree of bilateral loss was moderate, based on the quadratic mean (500Hz, 1000Hz, 2000Hz and 4000Hz). The mean post-fitting period until follow up was one month and three days. The average datalogged time of use is presented in Table 2.

Table 1. Characterization of the sample

Variables	n = 49 (35 elderly users and 14 non-elderly adult users)
Age (years) – average ± SD	66,0 ± 14,2
Minimum age/maximum age	24/91
Sex – n (%)	
Female	24(49,0)
Male	25(51,0)
Education (years) – median (P25 – P75)	6 (4 – 8)
Hearing aid use – n (%)	
Unilateral	8 (16,3)
Bilateral	41(83,7)
Period of adjustment to HA – average ± SD	33,6 ± 3,0
HHIE – S – median (P25 – P75)	6 (0 -10)
HHIE Classification– S – n (%)	
No participation restriction	24(68,6)
Slight to moderate participation restriction	9 (25,7)
Significant participation restriction	2(5,7)
HHIA – median (P25 – P75)	0 (0 - 15,5)
HHIA Classification– n (%)	
No participation restriction	11(78,6)
Slight participation restriction	1(7,1)
Moderate participation restriction	0(0,0)
Significant participation restriction	2 (14,3)
IOI-HA – average ± SD	29,3 ± 5,8

Legend: SD – standard deviation; % - percentage; HHIE – Hearing Handicap Inventory for Elderly-S – Screening version; HHIA – Hearing Handicap Inventory for Adult; IOI-HA = International Outcome Inventory for Hearing Aid; HA – Hearing Aids.

There was a significant negative correlation between the scores of the HHIE-S and IOI-HA questionnaires, showing that the greater the self-reported benefit and satisfaction, the lower the perception of restriction in social participation due to hearing loss. There was no significant correlation between the scores of the HHIA and IOI-HA questionnaires, nor was there a correlation between the scores of the questionnaires and the objective measures of HA time of use (Table 3).

Table 2. Patient hearing data and hearing aid time of use registered by datalogging

Variables	Right ear (n = 48)	Left ear (n = 46)	p
Time of use in hours/day median (P25 – P75)	3 (2 – 7)	3 (1 – 7)	0,380
Type of hearing loss – n (%)			0,513
Sensorineural	36(78,3)	36(80,0)	
Conductive	2(4,3)	3(6,7)	
Mixed	8 (17,4)	6 (13,3)	
Degree of hearing loss – n (%)			0,214
High-frequency hearing loss	2(4,2)	1(2,2)	
Mild	16(33,3)	15(32,6)	
Moderate	28(58,3)	23(50,0)	
Severe	2(4,2)	5 (10,9)	
Profound	0(0,0)	2(4,3)	
Quadratic mean – mean ± SD	47,1 ± 15,4	51,5 ± 22,7	0,228

Legend: SD – standard deviation; n – absolute number; p – percentage.

An analysis of the variables of education, age, quadratic mean and type of hearing loss and the scores from the questionnaires showed that there was no significant correlation between most of them, except for the negative correlation between the age variable and the IOI-HA questionnaire. This would suggest that the older the hearing aid user, the lower the level of self-reported satisfaction/benefit (Table 4). There was also an association between the variable of sex and the HHIA questionnaire (p = 0.020), revealing that female subjects declared more restriction in social participation, even after fitting, when compared to the male subjects.

In our analysis, we observed a difference between self-reported time of hearing aid use and the time of use objectively measured by datalogging software (Table 5) (z = - 4,74). It should be noted that, for such an analysis, self-reported daily time of use was classified according to the scales used in the IOI-HA questionnaire (i.e., 'never', 'less than 1 h/day', '1 - 4 h/day', '4 - 8 h/day', '8 < h/day').

Table 3. Datalogged time of use and its relationship with subjective measures of hearing aid use (questionnaires)

Relationships	Correlation coefficient	p
HHIE – S and IOI-HA	- 0,635	< 0,001
HHIE – S and time of use RE	0,107	0,545
HHIE – S and time of use LE	0,145	0,428
HHIA and IOI-HA	- 0,240	0,410
HHIA and time of use RE	- 0,354	0,235
HHIA and time of use LE	- 0,087	0,799
IOI-HA and time of use RE	0,159	0,287
IOI-HA and time of use LE	0,152	0,331

Legend: RE – right ear; LE – left ear; HHIE-S – Hearing Handicap Inventory for Elderly – Screening Version; HHIA - Hearing Handicap Inventory for Adult; IOI-HA = International Outcome Inventory for Hearing Aids.

Table 4.

Relationships	HHIE – S	HHIA	IOI-HA
Education	r_s = - 0,060 (p = 0,731)	r_s = 0,033 (p = 0,910)	r_s = 0,211 (p = 0,146)
Age	r_s = 0,265 (p = 0,124)	r_s = - 0,078 (p = 0,792)	r = - 0,317 (p = 0,026)
Quadratic mean			
RE	r_s = 0,159 (p = 0,363)	r_s = 0,090 (p = 0,758)	r = - 0,121 (p = 0,409)
LE	r_s = 0,288 (p = 0,094)	r_s = 0,237 (p = 0,415)	r = 0,049 (p = 0,736)
Type of hearing loss			
RE	r_s = 0,084 (p = 0,644)	r_s = - 0,101 (p = 0,742)	r_s = - 0,064 (p = 0,667)
LE	r_s=0,237 (p = 0,177)	r_s = 0,430 (p = 0,124)	r_s = 0,120 (p = 0,428)

Legend: RE – right ear; LE – left ear; HHIE-S – Hearing Handicap Inventory for Elderly – Screening Version; HHIA - Hearing Handicap Inventory for Adult; IOI-HA = International Outcome Inventory for Hearing Aids.

In our analysis of education and hearing aid time of use, no relevant association was found, either for the right ear (r_s = 0.221 and = 0.135) or for the left ear (r_s = 0.241 and = 0.120). No association between age and time of use was observed, either for the RE ($r_s = 0.174 - 0.202$ p) or for the LE ($r_s = -0,213 = p\ 0.170$).

Table 5. Analysis of self-reported HA time of use and its relationship with datalogged time of use

	Never n (%)	Less than 1h/day n (%)	1 – 4 h/day n (%)	4 – 8 h/day n (%)	< 8h/day n (%)	Total n (%)
Never n (%)	0 (0)	0 (0)	0 (0)	0 (0)	0 (0)	0 (0)
Less than 1h/day n (%)	1 (2,05)	0 (0)	1 (2.05)	0 (0)	0 (0)	2 (4,1)
1 – 4 h/day n (%)	0 (0)	0 (0)	4 (8,2)	0 (0)	0 (0)	4 (8,2)
4 – 8 h/day n (%)	1 (2,05)	2 (4,1)	10 (20,4)	4 (8,2)	0 (0)	17 (34,7)
< 8h/day n (%)	0 (0)	1 (2,05)	12 (24,5)	2 (4,1)	11 (22,4)	26 (53,1)
Total n (%)	2 (4,1)	3 (6,15)	27 (55,1)	6 (12,2)	11 (22,4)	49 (100)

DISCUSSION

Population aging is currently one of the predominant themes in different fields, in Brazil and around the world. Senescence brings about physical changes that justify special health care for this population, which is rapidly changing the morphology of the Brazilian age pyramid [15, 16]. This fact would explain the large number of elderly patients in the present study sample, a reality which can also be corroborated by previously mentioned data concerning hearing loss. In that national health survey, the southern region of Brazil scored higher numbers of hearing loss handicap. Moreover, within this particular group, elderly adults constitute a higher proportion when compared with non-elderly adults [1].

On the other hand, the balance in patient sex observed in our study does not support findings in scientific literature that describe a greater demand for health care by female subjects [17]. The balance in the sample may be justified by the higher prevalence of men over 60 diagnosed with hearing loss, which has also been described in scientific literature [18].

Most of the sample consisted of subjects with lower levels of education or with an incomplete elementary education. This was expected due to the general social profile of the population attended at the university hospital [19]. This common factor among almost all sample participants prevented further analysis due to the homogeneous characteristic of this variable.

A predominant part of the subjects in our sample presented bilateral hearing loss, with the most prevalent type being sensorineural moderate loss. No significant difference between ears was observed. These data confirm those described in specialized literature [20]. During the fitting process, hearing aids were adapted in accordance with the characteristics of hearing loss presented by each patient in the sample. Most were fitted bilaterally, which benefits patients with hearing loss since it better facilitates sound localization and binaural summation, as well as better speech recognition in noisy environments [21].

We found no significant correlation between the results of the questionnaires used in the present study and the variables of schooling, age, quadratic mean and type of hearing loss, with the exception of the relationship between the IOI-HA questionnaire and the variable of age. This further substantiates findings in scientific literature that the older the HA user, the weaker the perception of satisfaction/benefit, since elderly individuals tend to understand age as a reason for disabilities. This general attitude might, therefore, make elderly HA users more demanding in terms of the satisfaction/benefit they expect from hearing aids [9].

Scores from questionnaires that measured self-reported restrictions in social participation or patient satisfaction/benefit in the post-fitting period were similar to those already found in specialized literature [9]. These results justify the negative correlation between the HHIE-S and the IOI-HA questionnaires. There was a significant correlation between the HHIA questionnaire and the variable of sex. Among non-elderly adults, follow-up self-reports revealed a greater perception of restriction in social participation. This may be explained by a stronger concern on the part of the adult female subjects for health issues, which may have influenced the results [17].

The non-association between questionnaire scores and datalogged time of use may be explained by the low average HA use by participants. This data may point to the need for closer and more frequent follow-ups for new users, in order to adjust and verify the adaptation process; two steps which have been referred to in the literature as important for better patient habituation to hearing aids [15]. It is important to note that, even with an average of three hours per day in the first month of adaptation, the subjects in this study predominantly reported benefit and satisfaction with their HAs. What is more, reports regarding restriction in social participation were mostly absent, both in elderly and non-elderly adults. This finding is also similar to those present in scientific literature [11]. It should be taken into account, however, that results may also have been influenced by the fact that these patients received their hearing aids through the unified public health system, at no financial cost to themselves.

The present study showed that sample subjects overestimated the average daily time of use of the hearing aids in their self-report. This finding corroborates previous research [22], in which there was also overestimation in the self-reported time of use of hearing devices; however, the study group was smaller than the sample in this study. It is worth noting that data may reflect certain characteristics of the each sample, since in another study no overestimation in self-reports of sample subjects was observed when compared to the time of use provided by datalogging [13].

It is important to highlight that our study was carried out with participants whose health evaluations and care are provided by a unified public health system. This fact, in turn, probably influenced results with respect to patient perception of time of use, satisfaction/benefit and restriction in social participation. Apart from this, lower levels of education may have compromised patient understanding of the need for hearing aids, as well as instructions regarding the proper handling and care of these devices. In like manner, the overestimated time of use in self-reports may correspond to certain characteristics of particular groups of users who may feel the need to declare increased times because of the way in which the hearing aids are distributed to the public.

Thus, our data show, above all, the need for improved guidance for patients attended at the hospital, taking into consideration the way in which hearing aids are made available to them (for example, via public funds), the need for continued use so that greater and better benefits can be obtained, as well as the relation between hearing and different aspects of daily life, especially social and cognitive ones.

CONCLUSION

Through questionnaires applied to the patient sample of the present study, we were able to verify that the majority of and elderly and non-elderly users fitted with hearing aids felt satisfied and considered the devices beneficial. Additionally, for the most part, responses revealed no significant restriction in social participation. However, no association was found between the questionnaires and the datalogged times of use. Nonetheless, there was a significant difference between question one of the IOI-HA questionnaire and datalogged times of use, suggesting an overestimation in the self-reported time of use of hearing aids by patients. There was a negative correlation between the HHIE-S and IOI-HA questionnaires. This brings to the fore the important relationship between patients self-reporting no restriction in social participation as well as satisfaction and benefit after being fitted with hearing aids.

REFERENCES

[1] Brazilian Institute of Geography and Statistics. *National Health Survey 2013: Life Cycles*. Brasil, 2013.

[2] Cruz, Mariana S., Oliveira, Luiz R., Carandina, Luana, Lima, Maria Cristina P., César, Chester Luiz G., Barros, Marilisa B. A., Alves, Maria Cecília G. P. & Goldbaum, Moises. (2009). Prevalence of self-reported hearing loss and attributed causes: a population-based study.

Cadernos de Saúde Pública, 25, 1123-31. Accessed December 18, 2018. doi: 10.1590/S0102-311X2009000500019.

[3] Teixeira, Adriane R., Almeida, Luciane., Jotz, Geraldo P. & De Barba, Marion. (2008). Quality of life of adults and elderly people after hearing aids adaptation. *Revista da Sociedade Brasileira de Fonoaudiologia*, *13*, 357-61.

[4] Ministério, da Saúde. (2004). *Portaria 589* (National Politics of Hearing Health). Ministério da Saúde. Accessed in November 25, 2018. http://bvsms.saude.gov.br/bvs/saudelegis/sas/2004/prt0589_08_10_2004_rep.html.

[5] Ministério, da Saúde. (2011). *Portaria 793* (Network of care for people with disabilities under the Unified Health System). Accessed in November 25, 2018. http:// bvsms.saude.gov.br/bvs/saudelegis/ gm/2012/prt0793_24_04_2012.html.

[6] Ferraz, Tatiane N., Sant'Ana, Erika S. N., Mazini, Jéssica B. & Scharlach, Renata C. (2015). Verification and Validation Procedures in the Individual Hearing Aid Selection and Fitting Process: Choices of the Audiologists. *Revista Equilíbrio Corporal e Saúde*, *6*, 40-7. Accessed in November 30, 2018. http://www.pgsskroton.com.br/ seer/index.php/reces/article/view/2442.

[7] Broca, Vanessa S. & Scharlach, Renata C. (2014). The use of self-assessment questionnaires for validation of the results in hearing aid selection and fitting process. *Revista CEFAC*, *16*, 1808-19. Accessed in December, 30, 2018. doi: 10.1590/1982-0216201410513.

[8] Silva, Deide P. C. B., Silva, Virginia B. & Aurélio, Fernanda S. (2013). Auditory Satisfaction of patients fitted with hearing aids in the Brazilian Public Health Service and benefit offered by the hearing aids. *Brazilian Journal of Otorhinolaryngology*, *79*, 538-45. Accessed in December 30, 2018. doi: 10.5935/1808-8694.20130098.

[9] Grossi, Letícia M. R. & Scharlach, Renata C. (2011). Satisfaction and Participation restriction in hearing aids' users: a study with elderly. *Revista Equilíbrio Corporal e Saúde*, *3*, 3-15. Accessed in December 30, 2018. http://www.pgsskroton.com.br/seer/index.php/reces/article/ view/44/3147.

[10] Cox, Robin M. & Alexander, Genevieve C. (2002). The International Outcome Inventory for Hearing Aids (IOI-HA): psychometric properties of the English version. *International Journal of Audiology*, *41*, 30-5.

[11] Moda, Isabela., Mantello, Erika B., Reis, Ana Claudia M. B., Isaac, Myriam L., Oliveira, Andreia A. & Hyppolito, Miguel Angelo. (2013). Evaluation of hearing aid user satisfaction. *Revista CEFAC*, *15*, 778-85. Accessed in December 12, 2018. doi: 10.1590/S1516-18462013000400006.

[12] Laperuta, Erika B. & Fiorini, Ana Claudia. (2012). Satisfaction of elderly individuals with hearing aids in the first six months of use. *Jornal Sociedade Brasileira de Fonoaudiologia*, *24*, 316-21. Accessed in December 30, 2018. https://www.researchgate.net/publication/234104774_Satisfaction_of_elderly_individuals_with_hearing_aids_in_the_first_six_months_of_use.

[13] Makan, Aarti. (2015). *The value of using the Operational Model of behaviour change on adultaural rehabilitation outcomes.* MD diss., University of Pretoria.

[14] Souza, Valquiria C. & Lemos, Stela Maris. (2015). Tools for evaluation of restriction on auditory participation: systematic review of the literature. *CoDAS*, *27*, 400-6. Accessed in December 30, 2018. doi: 10.1590/2317-1782/20152015008.

[15] Mondelli, Maria Fernanda C. G. & Silva, Letícia L. (2011). Profile of the Patients Serviced in a High Complexity System. *Arquivos Internacionais de. Otorrinolaringologia*, *15*, 29-34. Accesssed in December 20, 2018. doi: 10.1590/S1809-48722011000100004.

[16] Silva, Alexandre M. M., Mambrini, Juliana V. M., Peixoto, Sergio V., Malta, Deborah C. & Lima-Costa, Maria Fernanda. (2017). Use of health services by Brazilian elderly with and without functional limitation. *Revista de Saúde Pública*, *51*, 1-10. Accessed in December 20, 2018. doi: 10.1590/s1518-8787.2017051000243.

[17] Vieira, Katiuscia L. D., Gomes, Vera Lúcia O., Borba, Marta R. & Costa, César Francisco S. (2013). Health care for male population in basic unit of family health: reasons for (not) attendance. *Escola Anna*

Nery Revista de Enfermagem, 17, 120-7. Accessed in December 30, 2018. doi: 10.1590/S1414-81452013000100017.

[18] Petry, T. (2007). *Epidemiological profile of the patients treated at the hearing aid laboratory of the Federal University of Santa Maria.* Specialization monograph., Universidade Federal de Santa Maria.

[19] Picinini, Taís A., Weigert, Liese L., Neves, Camila Z. & Teixeira, Adriane R. (2017). Restriction of social participation and satisfaction of hearing aids - post-adaptation study. *Audiology Communication Research, 22*, 1-8. Accessed in December 30, 2018. doi:10.1590/2317-6431-2016-1830.

[20] Baraldi, Giovana S., Almeida, Lais C. & Borges, Alda C. C. (2007). Hearing loss in aging. *Revista Brasileira de Otorrinolaringologia, 73*, 64-70. Accessed in December 30, 2018. http://www.scielo.br/pdf/rboto/v73n1/a10v73n1.pdf.

[21] Mueller, Gustav H., Ricketts, Todd. & Bentler, Ruth. (2014). *Modern hearing aids: pre-fitting testing and selection considerations.* San Diego, Plural.

[22] Gaffney, Patricia. (2008). Reported hearing aid use versus datalogging in a VA population. *Hearing Review, 15*, 42. Accessed in December 30, 2018. http://www.hearingreview.com/2008/06/reported-hearing-aid-use-versus-datalogging-in-a-va-population/.

In: Advances in Audiology Research
Editor: Victor M. Kristensen

ISBN: 978-1-53615-260-9
© 2019 Nova Science Publishers, Inc.

Chapter 4

POSTUROLOGY: THE SCIENTIFIC INVESTIGATION OF POSTURAL DISORDERS

Giuseppe Messina[1,2], MD, Valerio Giustino[3], Francesco Dispenza[4,5], MD, PhD, Francesco Galletti[6], Angelo Iovane[1], MD, Serena Rizzo[7], MD and Francesco Martines[5,8,*], MD, PhD

[1]Department of Psychology,
Educational Science and Human Movement,
University of Palermo, Palermo, Italy
[2]PosturaLab Italia Research Institute, Palermo, Italy
[3]PhD Program in Health Promotion and Cognitive Sciences,
University of Palermo, Palermo, Italy
[4]A.O.U.P. Paolo Giaccone, Palermo, Italy
[5]Istituto Euromediterraneo di Scienza e Tecnologia – IEMEST,
Palermo, Italy
[6]Department of Otorhinolaryngology,
University of Messina, Messina, Italy

---

* Corresponding Author's E-mail: francescomartines@hotmail.com

[7]Di.Chir.On.S. Department, Physical medicine and rehabilitation,
University of Palermo, Palermo, Italy
[8]Bio.Ne.C. Department, Audiology Section,
University of Palermo, Palermo, Italy

ABSTRACT

The human posture, regulated by the tonic postural system in response to the phenomenon of the force of gravity, is organized by feedback and feedforward processes according to a non-linear cybernetic system in which the central nervous system integrates sensory inputs from interoceptive, proprioceptive and exteroceptive organs modulating the muscular tone. According to this scheme, afferences from sensory organs such as the muscular proprioceptors organs, the stomatognathic apparatus, the visual system as well as the auditory and the vestibular system are responsible for controlling balance and postural control. If one of these postural receptors is dysfunctional (i.e., it does not function physiologically), it sends aberrant informations to the central nervous system, which modulates a response that generates an adaptation of the muscular tone through muscle chains according to a non-linear dynamic relationship. The posturography, comprising the baropodometric evaluation and the stabilometric assessment, is an instrumental evaluation that allows, through a platform, to measure body posture. In particular, pressure and plantar surface contribute to provide fundamental postural characteristics, whereas, the study of the centre of pressure (i.e., the point of the load pressure sum of the ground reaction force vector) is used to evaluate body balance and postural control.

The purpose of this chapter is to understand the main features of human posture and how it is possible to analyze it.

Keywords: posture, stability, body balance

INTRODUCTION

The Posturology is the science that studies human posture in static and dynamic and the relationship existing between body segments. The human posture can be represented as a non-linear cybernetic system that is regulated by the tonic postural system, antigravity musculature which allows to control body stability subject to the force of gravity. Indeed, the muscle apparatus maintains a basal activity, called tone, in order to react to the force of gravity without performing changing on physical location or movements of skeletal parts of human body [1].

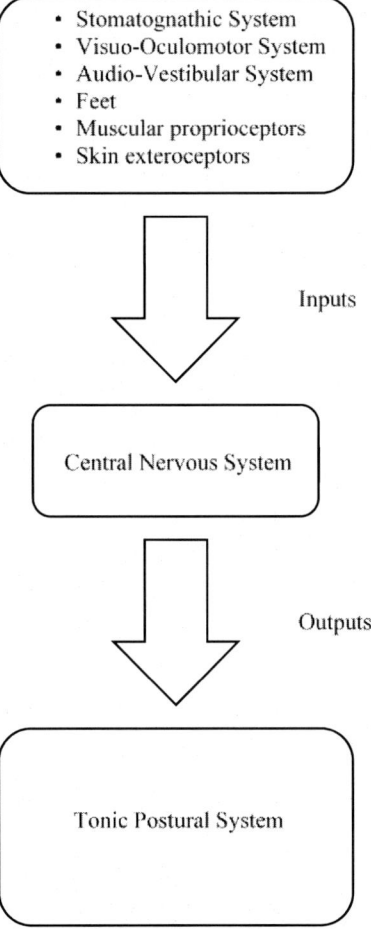

Figure 1. The non-linear cybernetic system of the human posture.

Body posture is influenced by afferents from sensory receptors as the stomatognathic system, the visual apparatus, the audio-vestibular system, the feet, the muscular proprioceptors organs, the skin [2-8]. As represented in the Figure 1, these organs project sensory information into the central nervous system that integrates the afferents and processes a response to the tonic postural system [1]. A change in the inputs from these systems due to a physiological decline or a pathological condition causes adaptation mechanism through the muscle chains causing altered effects on body balance [9-14]. Moreover, it is important to note that, according to the non-linear dynamic relationship, cause and effect could not correspond in terms of proportion and for a small phenomenon could be present a major consequence.

In case of altered sensory information from a postural receptor the tonic postural system responds changing muscular activity modulating the tone leading adaptation mechanisms as long as it is possible until the postural disorder.

The role of the posturologist is to evaluate body balance and posture features, in qualitative and quantitative manner, in order to understand the cause of a possible postural disorder.

HUMAN POSTURE EVALUATION

Body posture assessment comprehends: patient history acquisition, visual postural analysis, postural clinical tests and the posturography (including baropodometric assessment and the stabilometric assessment).

PATIENT HISTORY

An accurate patient history obtainment facilitates the identification of the cause of the postural disorder. Accordingly, the inquiry should provide elements of knowledge about: trauma, accidents, injuries as well as previous surgical operations, allergies/intolerances, pains but also diseases/impairments and/or taking drugs, treatments in progress, sight or hearing loss, audiovestibular characteristics as the presence of tinnitus, vertigo/dizziness, aural fullness [15-22]. Furthermore, the posturologist should collect data regarding lifestyle features as sleep quality, stress or anxiety state, physical activity level and type of job, important contributors that determine human posture [23-29]. Moreover, it was widely investigated in the literature the role of occlusal or orthopedic devices on human posture, for this reason for the expert in posturology it is important to annotate also these informations [30-32].

VISUAL POSTURAL ANALYSIS

The observation of the posture is an essential part of the body posture evaluation. This qualitative assessment take into consideration the spatial location of peculiar points of the body in order to analyze any deviations respect to the vertical line for the sagittal and the frontal plane and possible rotations in the horizontal plane [33]. Moreover, it is possible to examine the alignement of body segments and the differences between rightward and leftward hemibody [33].

For the visual postural analysis the subject is asked to maintain the orthostatic stance as comfortably as possible wearing only underwear, barefoot and looking forward while the posturologist records the location of the landmarks for all the anatomical planes as represented in the Figure 2a,b,c. In particular, in the frontal plane the following lines are considered: the bipupillary line, the connection line of acoustic meatus, the line connecting left and right labial commissures, the bi-acromial line, the bi-styloid line and the bi-ischial line (Figure 1). In absence of any postural disorder, all these reference lines should be parallel to each other. To assess postural features in the sagittal plane, the alignment of peculiar points passing through the vertical axis, i.e., the acoustic meatus, the odontoid process of the second cervical vertebra, the body of the third lumbar vertebra and the lateral malleolus, is taken into consideration (Figure 2a). Moreover, the cervical curve of the spine should measure 6 - 8 cm and the lumbar curve 4-6 cm. In the evaluation of the horizontal plane the main reference lines concern the parallelism between the shoulder girdle and the pelvic girdle (Figure 2c).

POSTURAL CLINICAL TESTS

Since, as mentioned above, all the postural receptors lead sensory information to the central nervous system influencing the tonic postural system, postural clinical tests are performed to identify a dysfunctional postural receptor. Indeed, these tests allow the evaluation of the physiological function of the organs involved on postural regulation. Among these assessments, it is important to mention the ocular motility exam, the swallowing evaluation and the vestibular function tests.

POSTUROGRAPHY

Posturography, or instrumental postural assessment, includes a baropodometric test, an examination that allows the measurement of the foot pressure and the plantar surface and a stabilometric test, for the measurement of the regulation of the activity of the postural tonic system. Posturography is measured using a platform that samples real time postural sway at different frequency based on the type of the platform.

The baropodometry is measured in 5 seconds during which the patient maintains the orthostatic position on the platform with the head in a neutral position facing forward, the arms along the trunk and the feet positioned next to each other. The main features measured through this test are the load distribution between feet, the rearfoot/forefoot ratio of the load pressure for each foot and the plantar surface characteristics.

The duration of the stabilometry is 51.2 seconds and provides that the subject mantains the feet positioned side-by-side and forming an angle of 30° and both heels at 4 cm apart [34].

Posturology: The Scientific Investigation of Postural Disorders

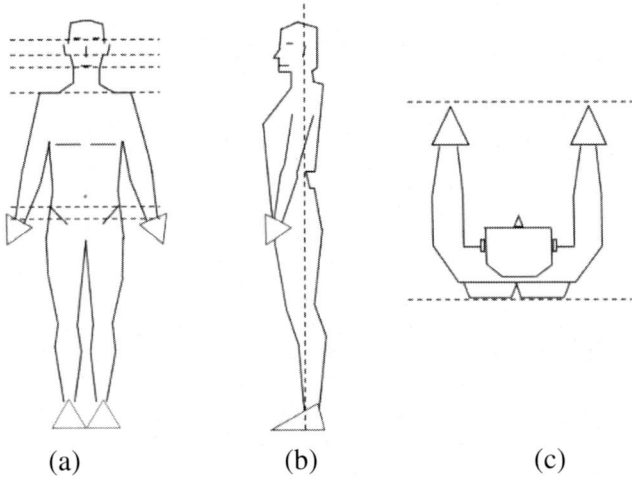

Figure 2a, b, c. The visual postural analysis in the frontal, sagittal and horizontal plane respectively.

Basic, participant repeate the stabilometric test in two different conditions: with eyes open and then with eyes closed to examine the impact of sight on posture. Moreover, complementary stabilometric tests are used to investigate the influence of all the others receptors on stability, such as the test with caloric vestibular stimulation for the vestibule or the stabilometric assessment with mouth open to evaluate the effect of the stomatognathic system on postural control [35,36]. In the Table 1 are illustrated some methods to analyze the influence of sensory information from postural organs on body balance. The parameters considered for the postural sway are the coordinates of the center of pressure (CoP) and in particular the Sway Path Length (SPL), i.e., the path length of the center of pressure, and the Ellipse Sway Area (ESA), i.e., the surface that contains the movement of the CoP.

INTERVENTION PROGRAMS

As mentioned previously, a postural disorder is caused by an altered postural receptor. For this reason, if the posturologist identifies a postural disorder by posture evaluation, the treatment to rebalance the system depends on which receptor is in dysfunction. Furthermore, intercepted the receptor, the intervention can provide a wide range of approaches.

Table 1. Some stabilometric tests for postural receptors

Visuo-Oculomotor System	With eyes closed With eyes towards different directions With prisms
Audio-Vestibular System	Caloric vestibular stimulation Galvanic vestibular stimulation
Stomatognathic System	With mouth open With occlusal splint

The role of the posturologist, in presence of a postural disorder, is to advise and direct the patient to visit the specialist (such as the gnathologist in case of swallowing disorder or the otorhinolaryngologist in presence of vertigo).

Anyhow, it is widely known that, within the various treatments proposed, physical activity is always recommended in order to improve balance [37].

REFERENCES

[1] Gagey, P. M. (1991). A critique of posturology: towards an alternative neuroanatomy?. *Surg Radiol Anat*, 13 (4): 255 - 257.

[2] Cuccia, A. & Caradonna, C. (2009). The relationship between the stomatognathic system and body posture. *Clinics (Sao Paulo)*, 64 (1): 61 - 66.

[3] Pociask, F. D., DiZazzo-Miller, R., Goldberg, A. & Adamo, D. E. (2016). Contribution of Head Position, Standing Surface, and Vision to Postural Control in Community-Dwelling Older Adults. *American Journal of Occupational Therapy*, 70 (1): 7001270010, 1-8.

[4] Thomas, E., Bianco, A., Messina, G., Mucia, M., Rizzo, S., Salvago, P., Sireci F., Palma, A. & Martines, F. (2017). The influence of

sounds in postural control. *Hearing Loss: Etiology, Management and Societal Implications*, 1 - 12.

[5] Martines, F., Messina, G., Patti, A., Battaglia, G., Bellafiore, M., Messina, A., Rizzo, S., Salvago, P., Sireci, F., Traina, M. & Iovane, A. (2015). Effects of tinnitus on postural control and stabilization: A pilot study. *Acta Medica Mediterranea*, 31: 907 - 912.

[6] Cobb, S. C., Bazett-Jones, D. M., Joshi, M. N., Earl-Boehm, J. E. & James, C. R. (2014). The relationship among foot posture, core and lower extremity muscle function, and postural stability. *Journal of Athletic Training*, 49 (2): 173 - 80.

[7] Li, S., Zhuang, C., Hao, M., He, X., Marquez, J. C., Niu, C. M. & Lan, N. (2015). Coordinated alpha and gamma control of muscles and spindles in movement and posture. *Frontiers in Computational Neuroscience*, 9: 122.

[8] Beaudette, S. M., Zwambag, D. P., Bent, L. R. & Brown, S. H. M. (2017). Spine postural change elicits localized skin structural deformation of the trunk dorsum in vivo. *Journal of the Mechanical Behavior of Biomedical Materials*, 67: 31 - 39.

[9] Whipple, R., Wolfson, L., Derby, C., Singh, D. & Tobin, J. (1993). Altered sensory function and balance in older persons. *Journal of Gerontology*, 48 Spec No: 71 - 76.

[10] Helbostad, J. L., Vereijken, B., Hesseberg, K. & Sletvold, O. (2009). Altered vision destabilizes gait in older persons. *Gait Posture*, 30 (2): 233 - 238.

[11] Thomas, E., Martines, F., Bianco, A., Messina, G., Giustino, V., Zangla, D., Iovane, A. & Palma, A. (2018). Decreased postural control in people with moderate hearing loss. *Medicine (Baltimore)*, 97 (14): e0244.

[12] Sung, P. S. & Maxwell, M. J. (2017). Kinematic chain reactions on trunk and dynamic postural steadiness in subjects with recurrent low back pain. *Journal of Biomechanics*, 59: 109 -115.

[13] Fortin, C., Feldman, D. E., Tanaka, C., Houde, M. & Labelle, H. (2012). Inter-rater reliability of the evaluation of muscular chains

associated with posture alterations in scoliosis. *BMC Musculoskeletal Disorders*, 13: 80.

[14] Hamaoui, A., Friant, Y. & Le Bozec, S. (2011). Does increased muscular tension along the torso impair postural equilibrium in a standing posture?. *Gait Posture*, 34 (4): 457 - 461.

[15] Salvago, P., Rizzo, S., Bianco, A. & Martines, F. (2017). Sudden sensorineural hearing loss: is there a relationship between routine haematological parameters and audiogram shapes?. *International Journal of Audiology*, 56 (3): 148 - 153.

[16] Scorpecci, A., Massoud, M., Giannantonio, S., Zangari, P., Lucidi, D., Martines, F., Foligno, S., Di Felice, G., Minozzi, A., Luciani, M. & Marsella, P. (2018). Otogenic lateral sinus thrombosis in children: proposal of an experience-based treatment flowchart. *Eur. Arch. Otorhinolaryngol.*, 275 (8): 1971 - 1977.

[17] Tjernström, F., Fransson, P. A., Holmberg, J., Karlberg, M. & Magnusson, M. (2009). Decreased postural adaptation in patients with phobic postural vertigo — an effect of an "anxious" control of posture?. *Neuroscience letters*, 454 (3): 198 - 202.

[18] Sasaki, O., Gagey, P. M., Ouaknine, A. M., Martinerie, J., Le Van Quyen, M., Toupet, M. & L'Heritier, A. (2001). Nonlinear analysis of orthostatic posture in patients with vertigo or balance disorders. *Neuroscience letters*, 41 (2): 185 - 192.

[19] Borel, L., Lopez, C., Péruch, P. & Lacour, M. (2008). Vestibular syndrome: a change in internal spatial representation. *Neurophysiol Clin.*, 38 (6): 375 - 389.

[20] Di Stadio, A., Dipietro, L., Toffano, R., Burgio, F., De Lucia, A., Ippolito, V., Garofalo, S., Ricci, G., Martines, F., Trabalzini, F. & Della Volpe, A. (2018). Working Memory Function in Children with Single Side Deafness Using a Bone-Anchored Hearing Implant: A Case-Control Study. *Audiol Neurootol*, 23 (4): 238 - 244.

[21] Kogler, A., Lindfors, J., Odkvist, L. M. & Ledin, T. (2000). Postural stability using different neck positions in normal subjects and patients with neck trauma. *Acta Otolaryngol.*, 120 (2): 151 - 155.

[22] Thomas, E., Ferrara, S., Messina, G., Passalacqua, M. I., Rizzo, S., Salvago, P., Palma, A. & Martines, F. (2017). The motor development of preterm infants after the neonatal intensive care unit. *Neonatal Intensive Care Units (NICUs): Clinical and Patient Perspectives, Levels of Care and Emerging Challenges.*

[23] Staab, J. P., Balaban, C. D. & Furman, J. M. (2013). Threat assessment and locomotion: clinical applications of an integrated model of anxiety and postural control. *Seminars in Neurology*, 33 (3): 297 - 306.

[24] Coco, M., Fiore, A. S., Perciavalle, V., Maci, T., Petralia, M. C., Perciavalle, V. (2015). Stress exposure and postural control in young females. *Molecular Medicine Reports*, 11 (3): 2135 - 2140.

[25] Barcellona, M., Giustino, V., Messina, G., Battaglia, G., Fischetti, F., Palma, A. & Iovane, A. (2018). Effects of a specific training protocol on posturographic parameters of a taekwondo elite athlete and implications on injury prevention: A case study. *Acta Medica Mediterranea*, 34: 1533 - 1538.

[26] Goulème, N., Gérard, C. L. & Bucci, M. P. (2015). The Effect of Training on Postural Control in Dyslexic Children. *PLoS One*, 10 (7): e0130196.

[27] Bellafiore, M., Battaglia, G., Bianco, A., Paoli, A., Farina, F. & Palma, A. (2011). Improved postural control after dynamic balance training in older overweight women. *Aging Clinical and Experimental Research*, 23 (5-6): 378 - 385.

[28] Hlavenka, T. M., Christner, V. F. K. & Gregory, D. E. (2017). Neck posture during lifting and its effect on trunk muscle activation and lumbar spine posture. *Applied Ergonomics*, 62: 28 - 33.

[29] Caneiro, J. P., O'Sullivan, P., Burnett, A., Barach, A., O'Neil, D., Tveit, O. & Olafsdottir, K. (2010). The influence of different sitting postures on head/neck posture and muscle activity. *Manual Therapy*, 15 (1): 54 - 60.

[30] Battaglia, G., Giustino, V., Iovane, A., Bellafiore, M., Martines, F., Patti, A., Traina, M., Messina, G. & Palma, A. (2016). Influence of

occlusal vertical dimension on cervical spine mobility in sports subjects. *Acta Medica Mediterranea*, 32: 1589 - 1595.

[31] De Giorgi, I., Castroflorio, T., Cugliari, G. & Deregibus, A. (2018). Does occlusal splint affect posture? A randomized controlled trial. *Cranio*, 1 - 9.

[32] Kendall, J. C., Bird, A. R. & Azari, M. F. (2014). Foot posture, leg length discrepancy and low back pain — their relationship and clinical management using foot orthoses — an overview. *Foot (Edinb)*, 24 (2): 75 - 80.

[33] Ferreira, E. A., Duarte, M., Maldonado, E. P., Bersanetti, A. A., Marques, A. P. (2011). Quantitative assessment of postural alignment in young adults based on photographs of anterior, posterior, and lateral views. *J Manipulative Physiol Ther*, 34 (6): 371 - 380.

[34] Scoppa, F., Gallamini, M., Belloni, G. & Messina, G. (2017). Clinical stabilometry standardization: Feet position in the static stabilometric assessment of postural stability. *Acta Medica Mediterranea*, 33: 707 - 713.

[35] Rode, G., Tiliket, C., Charlopain, P., Boisson D. (1998). Postural asymmetry reduction by vestibular caloric stimulation in left hemiparetic patients. *Scand J Rehabil Med*, 30 (1): 9 - 14.

[36] Ohlendorf, D., Riegel, M., Lin Chung, T., Kopp, S. (2013). The significance of lower jaw position in relation to postural stability. Comparison of a premanufactured occlusal splint with the Dental Power Splint. *Minerva Stomatol*, 62 (11 - 12): 409 - 417.

[37] Whitney, S. L., Alghwiri, A., Alghadir, A. (2015). Physical therapy for persons with vestibular disorders. *Curr Opin Neurol*, 28 (1): 61 - 68.

In: Advances in Audiology Research
Editor: Victor M. Kristensen

ISBN: 978-1-53615-260-9
© 2019 Nova Science Publishers, Inc.

Chapter 5

THE INFLUENCE OF OTOVESTIBULAR SYSTEM ON BODY POSTURE

Francesco Martines[1,2,*], *MD, PhD, Valerio Giustino*[3], *Francesco Dispenza*[1,4], *MD, PhD, Francesco Galletti*[5], *Angelo Iovane*[6], *MD, Serena Rizzo*[7], *MD and Giuseppe Messina*[6,8], *MD.*

[1]Istituto Euromediterraneo di Scienza e Tecnologia – IEMEST, Palermo, Italy
[2]Bio.Ne.C. Department, Audiology Section, University of Palermo, Palermo, Italy
[3]PhD Program in Health Promotion and Cognitive Sciences, University of Palermo, Palermo, Italy
[4]A.O.U.P. Paolo Giaccone, Palermo, Italy
[5]Department of Otorhinolaryngology, University of Messina, Messina, Italy

---

* Corresponding Author's E-mail: francescomartines@hotmail.com.

[6]Department of Psychology,
Educational Science and Human Movement,
University of Palermo, Palermo, Italy
[7]Di. Chir.On.S. Department, Physical medicine and rehabilitation,
University of Palermo, Palermo, Italy
[8]PosturaLab Italia Research Institute, Palermo, Italy

Abstract

It is well-known that body posture is controlled by an integration, at the level of the central nervous system, of afferences coming from various organs that influences the tonic postural system responsible for the alignment of the skeletal body segment of the human body, for balance and for postural control. Many studies have shown that the auditory and the vestibular systems contribute significantly to posture. The scientific literature reported that patients suffering from hearing impairment or vestibular disorders may be affected by loss of balance or inability to maintain postural control. Furthermore, many researchers have demonstrated a significant correlation between hearing loss and the risk of falling. Non-physiological sensory information from the otovestibular system negatively interferes on posture inducing asymmetrical muscular tensions that determines postural disorders. In these patients, a postural sway analysis, using a stabilometric platform, and a gait analysis, through a dynamic baropodometric test, can be considered in order to measure their ability to maintain static and dynamic balance and to examine their potential improvement after an otovestibular rehabilitation. The aim of this work is to investigate the influence of hearing loss and vestibular disorders on body posture.

Keywords: body balance, vestibular disorders, hearing loss

The Otovestibular System

Among the sensory organs, the otovestibular apparatus represents a complex system able to project to the central nervous system the sensory information concerning auditory, sense of position, and perception of movement in the space of the head in order to regulate approppriately static and dynamic body balance [1].

The cochlea is an auditory organ responsible for the transduction of mechanical waves into electrical signals that reach the central nervous system (CNS) through the cochlear nerve. Regarding the vestibular component, the afferents from this apparatus are integrated at the level of the central nervous system (CNS) in addition to the visuo-oculomotor and proprioceptive information. Consequently, the CNS produces efferent responses to the ocular muscles and the spinal cord, generating the vestibulo-ocular reflex (VOR) and the vestibulospinal reflex (VSR). The latter generates compensatory movements in order to regulate and maintain body balance, the former movements of the oculomotor muscles in base of changing head positions [1]. Both reflexes are fundamental to adjust and control body balance.

The cochlea as well as the vestibule are located in the inner ear and both sensory information coming from these organs influences human posture [2-6].

OTOVESTIBULAR SENSORY INFORMATIONS

Although it is well-known that all the sensory systems contribute to the regulation of posture and to the maintenance of balance, a physiological prevalence of discernment of sensory informations in correlation with age exists [7]. In particular, at birth, body posture depends mainly on labyrinthic and sound stimuli, whereas when the human being adopts a bipedal stance, the static postural control is managed above all by proprioceptive inputs from the foot and the paravertebral muscles instead, and for the dynamic postural control, from visual afferences. However, the scientific literature has demonstrated the importance of audio-vestibular sensory information on body posture in children as well as in elderly [8-12].

OTOVESTIBULAR DISORDERS AND BODY BALANCE

As the regulation of the activity of the tonic postural system and the abilty to maintain body balance depends on all the sensory postural receptors, a physiological decline of the audio-vestibular system, hearing impairment, or vestibular disorders affect body balance [13-17]. In particular, hearing loss, the most common sensorial deterioration, has disadvantageous effects on the life quality and, among the adverse consequences, causes a possible alteration on body balance increasing the risk of falling especially in the elderly [18-21]. Likewise, it is widely recognized that, vestibular disorers such as tinnitus, vertigo, or dizziness have a significant impact on physiological and vital functions, and moreover, negatively influence postural control [16, 22-25].

In patients with damaging/disease of a sensory organ, the use of assistive devices, such as hearing aids or cochlear implants for the audio-vestibular system, can improve daily activities and, in general, the quality of life [8, 26, 27].

POSTUROGRAPHY: A QUANTITATIVE ASSESSMENT OF BODY BALANCE

The posturography allows the measurement of muscular activity of the tonic postural system. In these patients, this instrumental postural assessment is fundamental in order to measure their ability to maintain static and dynamic balance, and moreover, to examine any change after an otovestibular rehabilitation or a cochlear implant surgery [27-30]. In particular, by means of a baropodometric platform, it is possible to evaluate postural sway analysis, through a stabilometric test, and a gait analysis, through a dynamic baropodometric test [31].

Through the stabilometry it is possible to analyze the statokinesigram graph, i.e., the path of the center of pressure (CoP) and the surface that contains the movement of the CoP (the Sway Path Length (SPL) and the

Ellipse Sway Area (ESA) respectively), and the stabilogram graph that shows the CoP displacement during the time distinguished by direction (backwards/forwards and medial/lateral sway).

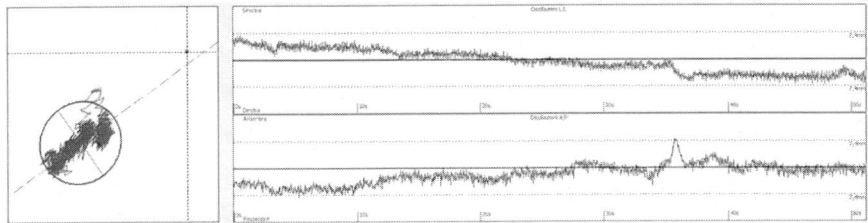

Figure 1. Statokinesigram (on the left) and stabilogram (on the right) of the stabilometric test. http://posturografia.it/wp-content/uploads/2017/04/posturografia_11.jpg.

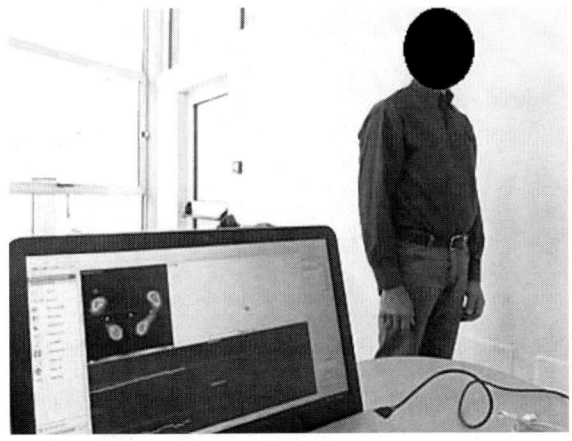

Figure 2. Stabilometric test.

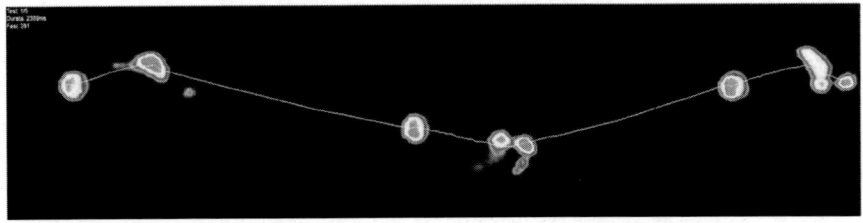

Figure 3. Study of the gait analysis through a dynamic baropodometric test http://pedanabaropodometrica.it/wp-content/uploads/2017/05/pedanabaropodometrica_10.jpg.

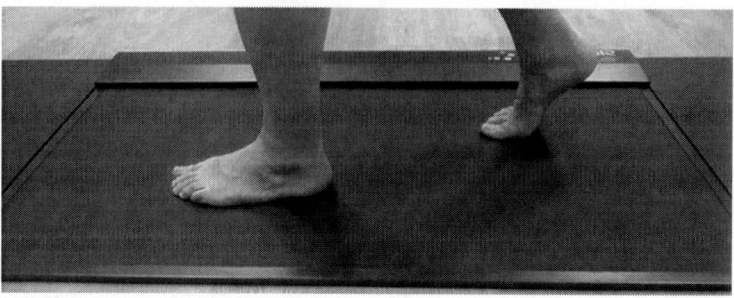

Figure 4. Baropodometric test https://www.sensormedica.com/site/images/pedana_120_50.jpg.

As sensitive and specific measures are a priority in order to detect vestibular disorders, Di Fabio has investigate the sensitivity and specificity of static and dinamic posturography to identify these patients [32]. The author shows that the posturography, if applied in isolation, turns out to be ineffective, in terms of sensitivity, to detect vestibular impairment. However, the association of posturography with the other vestibular function tests increased the sensitivity of identifying vestibular deficits from 61% to 89%.

INFLUENCE OF OTOVESTIBULAR SYSTEM ON BODY BALANCE

Many authors have investigated the impact of auditory stimuli, in terms of frequency, intensity, as well as sound duration, on body balance and the relationship between hearing loss and the risk of fall [7, 10, 14, 20, 21, 27, 29].

Although Mainenti et al. reported no significant differences on stabilometric parameters when subjects were submitted to different types of sound stimulation [33], contrarily, Raper and Soames [34] showed higher sway in sound conditions compared with no sound condition, with frequency stimulations at 250 Hz. In addition, a study by Park et al. reported that the Sway Path Length on the anterior-posterior axis increased with higher frequencies of sound [35]. Siedlecka et al. suggested that sound stimuli with frequencies from 1000 Hz to 4000 Hz influence cody stability [3].

Many studies have examined the role of sound intensity on body posture and the results seems to indicate that sound intensity higher than 90 dB affects postural stability [3, 36].

As reported in the scientific literature, sound duration affects body sway [33, 37, 38]. In particular, Kapoula et al. performed a stabilometry for 51.2 seconds finding a significant affect of sound disturbances on postural sway in patients with highly modulated tinnitus [37]. Contrariwise, many researches reported no significant influence when the stabilometric tests were performed for 20 or 30 seconds [33, 38].

THE ROLE OF PHYSICAL ACTIVITY ON BODY BALANCE

The scientific literature reported that, among the intrinsic factors, falls are related to the physiological decline of hearing, hearing impairments and vestibular disorders [39]. It is well-known that, among the treatments, exercise improves balance ability that induces a consequent fall reduction, and proves to be an effective intervention of falls prevention, in particular for older people [40, 41, 42]. The literature seems to be in agreement that balance exercises appears to be the most efficacious type of physical activity in order to improve body stability [43].

REFERENCES

[1] Spasiano, R., Mira, E. (2005). Anatomia e fisiologia del sistema vestibolare[Anatomy and physiology of the vestibular system]. *Clinica delle labirintopatie periferiche*, 45 - 64.

[2] Zhong, X., Yost, W. A. (2013). Relationship between postural stability and spatial hearing. *J Am Acad Audiol*, 24 (9): 782 - 788.

[3] Siedlecka, B., Sobera, M., Sikora, A., Drzewowska, I. (2015). The influence of sounds on posture control. *Acta Bioeng Biomech*, 17 (3): 96 - 102.

[4] Sakellari, V., Soames, R. W. (1996). Auditory and visual interactions in postural stabilization. *Ergonomics*, 39 (4): 634 - 648.

[5] Lopez, C. (2015). Making Sense of the Body: the Role of Vestibular Signals. *Multisens Res*, 28 (5-6): 525 - 557.

[6] Guerraz, M., Day, B. L. (2005). Expectation and the vestibular control of balance. *J Cogn Neurosci*, 17 (3): 463 - 469.

[7] Thomas, E., Bianco, A., Messina, G., Mucia, M., Rizzo, S., Salvago, P., Sireci F., Palma, A. and Martines, F. (2017). The influence of sounds in postural control. *Hearing Loss: Etiology, Management and Societal Implications*, 1 - 12.

[8] Ebrahimi, A. A., Movallali, G., Jamshidi, A. A., Haghgoo, H. A., Rahgozar, M. (2016). Balance Performance of Deaf Children With and Without Cochlear Implants. *Acta Med Iran*, 54 (11): 737 - 742.

[9] Huang, M. W., Hsu, C. J., Kuan, C. C., Chang, W. H. (2011). Static balance function in children with cochlear implants. *Int J Pediatr Otorhinolaryngol*, 75 (5): 700 - 703.

[10] Thomas, E., Martines, F., Bianco, A., Messina, G., Giustino, V., Zangla, D., Iovane, A., Palma, A. (2018). Decreased postural control in people with moderate hearing loss. *Medicine (Baltimore)*, 97 (14): e0244.

[11] Davis, A., McMahon, C. M., Pichora-Fuller, K. M., Russ, S., Lin, F., Olusanya, B. O., Chadha, S., Tremblay, K. L. (2016). Aging and Hearing Health: The Life-course Approach. *Gerontologist*, 56 Suppl 2: S 256 - 267.

[12] Criter, R. E., Honaker, J. A. (2017). Fall risk screening protocol for older hearing clinic patients. *Int J Audiol*, 56 (10): 767 - 774.

[13] Melo Rde, S., Lemos, A., Macky, C. F., Raposo, M. C., Ferraz, K. M. (2015). Postural control assessment in students with normal hearing and sensorineural hearing loss. *Braz J Otorhinolaryngol*, 81 (4): 431 - 438.

[14] Rumalla, K., Karim, A. M., Hullar, T. E. (2015). The effect of hearing aids on postural stability. *Laryngoscope*, 125 (3): 720 - 723.

[15] Martines, F., Messina, G., Patti, A., Battaglia, G., Bellafiore, M., Messina, A., Rizzo, S., Salvago, P., Sireci, F., Traina, M., Iovane, A. (2015). Effects of tinnitus on postural control and stabilization: A pilot study. *Acta Medica Mediterranea*, 31: 907 - 912.

[16] Schlick, C., Schniepp, R., Loidl, V., Wuehr, M., Hesselbarth, K., Jahn, K. (2016). Falls and fear of falling in vertigo and balance disorders: A controlled cross-sectional study. *J Vestib Res*, 25 (5-6): 241 - 251.

[17] Söhsten, E., Bittar, R. S., Staab, J. P. (2016). Posturographic profile of patients with persistent postural-perceptual dizziness on the sensory organization test. *J Vestib Res*, 26 (3): 319 - 326.

[18] Salvago, P., Rizzo, S., Bianco, A., Martines, F. (2017). Sudden sensorineural hearing loss: is there a relationship between routine haematological parameters and audiogram shapes? *International Journal of Audiology*, 56 (3): 148 - 153.

[19] Di Stadio, A., Dipietro, L., Toffano, R., Burgio, F., De Lucia, A., Ippolito, V., Garofalo, S., Ricci, G., Martines, F., Trabalzini, F., Della Volpe, A. (2018). Working Memory Function in Children with Single Side Deafness Using a Bone-Anchored Hearing Implant: A Case-Control Study. *Audiol Neurootol*, 23 (4): 238 - 244.

[20] Jiam, N. T., Li, C., Agrawal, Y. (2016). Hearing loss and falls: A systematic review and meta-analysis. *Laryngoscope*, 126 (11): 2587 - 2596.

[21] Agmon, M., Lavie, L., Doumas, M. (2017). The Association between Hearing Loss, Postural Control, and Mobility in Older Adults: A Systematic Review. *J Am Acad Audiol*, 28 (6): 575 - 588.

[22] Matsushima, J. I., Sakai, N., Ifukube, T. (1999). Effects of tinnitus on posture: a study of electrical tinnitus suppression. *Int Tinnitus J*, 5 (1): 35 - 39.

[23] Lin, H. W., Bhattacharyya, N. (2014). Impact of dizziness and obesity on the prevalence of falls and fall-related injuries. *Laryngoscope*, 124 (12): 2797 - 2801.

[24] Scorpecci, A., Massoud, M., Giannantonio, S., Zangari, P., Lucidi, D., Martines, F., Foligno, S., Di Felice, G., Minozzi, A., Luciani, M., Marsella, P. (2018). Otogenic lateral sinus thrombosis in children: proposal of an experience-based treatment flowchart. *Eur. Arch. Otorhinolaryngol.*, 275 (8): 1971 - 1977.

[25] Thomas, E., Ferrara, S., Messina, G., Passalacqua, M. I., Rizzo, S., Salvago, P., Palma, A., Martines, F. (2017). The motor development of preterm infants after the neonatal intensive care unit. Neonatal Intensive Care Units (NICUs): Clinical and Patient Perspectives, Levels of Care and Emerging Challenges.

[26] Battaglia, G., Giustino, V., Iovane, A., Bellafiore, M., Martines, F., Patti, A., Traina, M., Messina, G., Palma, A. (2016). Influence of occlusal vertical dimension on cervical spine mobility in sports subjects. *Acta Medica Mediterranea*, 32: 1589 - 1595.

[27] Shayman, C. S., Earhart, G. M., Hullar, T. E. (2017). Improvements in Gait With Hearing Aids and Cochlear Implants. *Otol Neurotol*, 38 (4): 484 - 486.

[28] Whitney, S. L., Marchetti, G. F., Schade, A. I. (2006). The relationship between falls history and computerized dynamic posturography in persons with balance and vestibular disorders. *Arch Phys Med Rehabil*, 87 (3): 402 - 407.

[29] Soto-Varela, A., Gayoso-Diz, P., Rossi-Izquierdo, M., Faraldo-García, A., Vaamonde-Sánchez-Andrade, I., del-Río-Valeiras, M., Lirola-Delgado, A., Santos-Pérez, S. (2015). Reduction of falls in older people by improving balance with vestibular rehabilitation (ReFOVeRe study): design and methods. *Aging Clin Exp Res*, 27 (6): 841 - 848.

[30] Vitkovic, J., Le, C., Lee, S. L., Clark, R. A. (2016). The Contribution of Hearing and Hearing Loss to Balance Control. *Audiol Neurootol*, 21 (4): 195 - 202.

[31] Scoppa, F., Gallamini, M., Belloni, G., Messina, G. (2017). Clinical stabilometry standardization: Feet position in the static stabilometric assessment of postural stability. *Acta Medica Mediterranea*, 33: 707 - 713.

[32] Di Fabio, R. P. (1995). Sensitivity and specificity of platform posturography for identifying patients with vestibular dysfunction. *Phys Ther*, 75 (4): 290 - 305.

[33] Mainenti, M. R., De Oliveira, L. F., De Melo Tavares De Lima, M. A., Nadal, J. (2007). Stabilometric signal analysis in tests with sound stimuli. *Exp Brain Res*, 181 (2): 229 - 236.

[34] Raper, S. A., Soames, R. W. (1991). The influence of stationary auditory fields on postural sway behaviour in man. *Eur J Appl Physiol Occup Physiol*, 63 (5): 363 - 367.

[35] Park, S. H., Lee, K., Lockhart, T., Kim, S. (2011). Effects of sound on postural stability during quiet standing. *J Neuroeng Rehabil*, 8: 67.

[36] Tanaka, T., Kojima, S., Takeda, H., Ino, S., Ifukube, T. (2001). The influence of moving auditory stimuli on standing balance in healthy young adults and the elderly. *Ergonomics*, 44 (15): 1403 - 1412.

[37] Kapoula, Z., Yang, Q., Lê, T. T., Vernet, M., Berbey, N., Orssaud, C., Londero, A., Bonfils, P. (2011). Medio-lateral postural instability in subjects with tinnitus. *Front Neurol*, 2: 35.

[38] Alessandrini, M., Lanciani, R., Bruno, E., Napolitano, B., Di Girolamo, S. (2006). Posturography frequency analysis of sound-evoked body sway in normal subjects. *Eur Arch Otorhinolaryngol*, 263 (3): 248 - 252.

[39] Callis, N. (2016). Falls prevention: Identification of predictive fall risk factors. *Appl Nurs Res*, 29: 53 - 58.

[40] Battaglia, G., Bellafiore, M., Bianco, A., Paoli, A., Palma, A. (2010). Effects of a dynamic balance training protocol on podalic support in older women. Pilot Study. *Aging Clin Exp Res*, 22 (5-6): 406 - 411.

[41] Barcellona, M., Giustino, V., Messina, G., Battaglia, G., Fischetti, F., Palma, A., Iovane, A. (2018). Effects of a specific training protocol on posturographic parameters of a taekwondo elite athlete and implications on injury prevention: A case study. *Acta Medica Mediterranea*, 34: 1533 - 1538.

[42] Puccio, G., Giuffré, M., Piccione, M., Piro, E., Malerba V., Corsello. G. (2014) Intrauterine growth pattern and birthweight discordance in

twin pregnancies: a retrospective study. *Ital J Pediatr,* 40:43. doi: 10.1186/1824-7288-40-43

[43] Sherrington, C., Whitney, J. C., Lord, S. R., Herbert, R. D., Cumming, R. G., Close, J. C. (2008). Effective exercise for the prevention of falls: a systematic review and meta-analysis. *J Am Geriatr Soc,* 56 (12): 2234 - 2243.

In: Advances in Audiology Research ISBN: 978-1-53615-260-9
Editor: Victor M. Kristensen © 2019 Nova Science Publishers, Inc.

Chapter 6

AUDITORY BRAINSTEM RESPONSE AND FREQUENCY FOLLOWING RESPONSE IN PATIENTS WITH SICKLE CELL DISEASE

Adriana L. Silveira[1,], Adriane R. Teixeira[1,†], Christina M. Bittar[2], João Ricardo Friedrisch[2], Daniela P. Dall'Igna[2] and Sergio S. Menna Barreto[2]*

[1]Children and Adolescent Health Post Graduate Program, Universidade Federal do Rio Grande do Sul and Speech Therapy and Audiology Service, Hospital de Clínicas de Porto Alegre, Porto Alegre, Rio Grande do Sul, Brazil

[2]Health and Human Communication Department, Universidade Federal do Rio Grande do Sul and Speech Therapy and Audiology Service, Hospital de Clínicas de Porto Alegre, Porto Alegre, Rio Grande do Sul, Brazil

---

[*] Corresponding Author's E-mail: alsilveira@hcpa.edu.br.
[†] Corresponding Author's E-mail: adriane.teixeira@gmail.com.

Abstract

The aim of this study was to analyze the auditory brainstem response (ABR) and frequency following response (FFR) in patients diagnosed with Sickle Cell Disease (SCD) who were referred to the outpatient hemoglobinopathy clinic at a public hospital in southern Brazil. Fifty-four individuals aged between 6 and 24 years [mean age ± SD (years), 14.1 ± 4.6] were evaluated. Pure tone audiometry, high frequency tonal audiometry, tympanometry, and transient evoked otoacoustic emission for determination of peripheral normality were performed; the overall results indicted normal auditory thresholds in all individuals. Subsequently, electrophysiological evaluations including ABR and FFR were performed; the analysis of the ABR responses revealed an alteration in 88.9% of the individuals and that of FFR in 98.1%. The achievement of auditory thresholds within the normal range and presence of otoacoustic emissions enabled but did not guarantee excellence in the auditory pathway of the evaluated individuals.

Keywords: sickle cell disease, hearing, auditory evoked potentials, electrophysiology

Introduction

Sickle cell disease (SCD) is an inherited disease characterized by abnormality of the hemoglobin in the red blood cell. Hemoglobin is composed of proteins and iron which imparts a red color to the blood and allows the fixation of oxygen for transport to the cells of tissues and organs in the living organism. During periods of decreased oxygen tension in the red blood cell's environment, the abnormal hemoglobin content results in the transformation to a sickle cell pattern. The morphological and associated physiological changes drastically reduce the ability of the red blood cells to navigate and provide oxygen throughout the body [1].

The World Health Organization report indicates that SCD is a common disease, affecting approximately 5% of the world's population [2]. In Brazil, it is the most prevalent genetic disease, predominantly affecting individuals of Black/African ethnicity, with heterogeneous distribution among the regions. The diagnosis is made through the foot test on the 5th day of life [3]. The prevalence rate is approximately 6 to 10% in the north and northeast regions and at a lower rate of 2 and 3% in the south and southeast regions. The prevalence rate in Rio Grande do Sul is estimated at only 2% of the present population [4].

Due to the vaso-occlusive nature of SCD, there is potential for hearing damage. The relationship between SCD and peripheral hearing loss has been reported, but the studies reveal variable findings. Some reports have indicated that peripheral hearing loss is correlated with possible damage caused by low oxygenation of the cochlea in patients with vaso-occlusions through the disease [1, 5, 6]. Other reports have indicated that neurological symptoms could lead to central impairment [6, 7]. The discrepancies between studies could be due to the differences in audiological evaluation and incidence of hearing loss of 12 to 66% [6].

The auditory changes impact the individual's quality of life through the difficulty in analyzing sound information as well as overall communication impairment. There are no studies to investigate the speech-evoked ABR in this population; hence, research in this field is of interest.

This study aimed to analyze the ABR and FFR in patients diagnosed with SCD with normal peripheral auditory evaluation.

METHODS

This was an observational cross-sectional case series study of patients referred to the hemoglobinopathy outpatient clinic at a public hospital in Rio Grande do Sul, Brazil (southern region of the country). The study was approved by the Research Ethics Committee at the hospital where the study was developed (number 44486215000005327) and conducted under ethical principles that protect the rights, dignity, and well-being of the participants. Patients of the age group of 6 to 24 years were included. The exclusion criteria were the presence of clinically relevant comorbidities, quitting during the evaluation, and unilateral or bilateral peripheral hearing loss.

Table 1. Parameters and Range of Normality Considered for ABR and FFR

ABR		FFR	
Parameters Used			
Stimulus	click	Stimulus	syllable [da_40 ms]
Number of sweeps	2 cycles 2048	Number of sweeps	3 cycles 1000
Presentation	ipsilateral	Presentation	ipsilateral
Rate	27.7/s	Rate	11.1/s
Polarity	rarefied	Polarity	alternating
Window	12 ms	Window	60 ms
Intensity	80 dB	Intensity	80 dB
Gain	100	Gain	150
Low-pass filter	1.5 KHz	Low-pass filter	3.0 KHz
High-pass filter	100 Hz	High-pass filter	100 Hz
Rejection EEG	20%	Rejection EEG	30%
Range of Normality Considered			
Measure	Latency (ms)	Measure	Latency (ms)	Amplitude (mV)
Wave I	1.11-2.07			
Wave III	3.30-3.98	Wave V	6.11-7.11	0.16-0.46
Wave V	5.25-5.89	Wave A	6.83-8.19	(-0.27)–(-1.03)
Interpeak I-III	1.91-2.19	VA Complex	0.51-1.27	0.41-1.53
Interpeak III-V	1.91-1.95	Peak C	16.73-18.65	(-0.18)–(-0.54)
Interpeak I-V	3.48-4.48	Peak F	38.51-40.95	(-0.24)–(-0.62)

ms, milisecond; dB, decibel; Hz, hertz; µV, microvolt.

The sequence of evaluations was as follows: tonal threshold audiometry, high frequency tonal audiometry, tympanometry, transient evoked otoacoustic emission, ABR, and FFR (syllable /da/). Equipment used for the evaluations were: AC-40 (Interacoustics), AT235h (Interacoustics), Eclipse EP25 (Interacoustics), and SmpartEP (Intelligent Hearing Systems). The first four exams were used only to establish peripheral normality.

The parameters for obtaining recordings for both the uptake and range of normality for ABR and FFR are described in Table 1. The parameters were adapted from the equipment protocol [8] for ABR, and those of

Russo et al. [9] and Gonçalves [10] for FFR. To determine the range of normality, two standard deviations of each measurement were considered, except for those for the amplitude of Wave V and Peak F that considered only one deviation due to asymmetry of the distribution under neural conduction. The tracings were analyzed and sent to two audiologists for judgment of the demarcation of the waves.

RESULTS

We evaluated 54 patients with a medical diagnosis of SCD, with mean age of 14.1 years. The sample was distributed in three age groups: twelve years-old (17 subjects, 31.5%); 12 to 18 years-old (24 subjects, 44.4%); 18 to 24 years-old (13 subjects, 24.1%). Twenty-four male individuals (44.4%) and 30 female individuals (55.6%) participated.

The ABR with click stimulus revealed a change in 88.9% of the sample, and the increase of absolute latency of waves III and V and interpeak I-III were predominant. There were no significant differences between the latencies obtained between the bilateral ears (Table 2); however, there was greater impairment in the male individuals and age group of 12 to 18 years-old (Table 3).

Table 2. Comparison of ABR results between the bilateral ears

Variables	Right Ear	Left Ear	p
	Mean ± SD	Mean ± SD	
Wave I	1.78 ± 0.10	1.76 ± 0.14	0.167
Wave III	3.98 ± 0.16	3.98 ± 0.18	0.873
Wave V	5.90 ± 0.20	5.90 ± 0.17	0.844
I-III	2.20 ± 0.16	2.21 ± 0.17	0.303
III-V	1.92 ± 0.11	1.92 ± 0.09	0.931
I-V	4.12 ± 0.20	4.14 ± 0.19	0.365

SD, standard deviation.

Table 3. Comparison of changes in ABR results according to sex and age group

Variables	Ears	Total Sample n (%)	Female n (%)	Male n (%)	p
click					
Wave I	Right	1 (1.9)	0 (0.0)	1 (4.2)	0.444
	Left	3 (5.6)	2 (6.7)	1 (4.2)	1.000
Wave III	Right	26 (48.1)	11 (36.7)	15 (62.5)	0.107
	Left	23 (42.6)	9 (30.0)	14 (58.3)	0.069
Wave V	Right	31 (57.4)	12 (40.0)	19 (79.2)	0.009
	Left	28 (51.9)	13 (43.3)	15 (62.5)	0.260
I-III	Right	30 (55.6)	11 (36.7)	19 (79.2)	0.004
	Left	35 (64.8)	15 (50.0)	20 (83.3)	0.024
III-V	Right	18 (33.3)	7 (23.3)	11 (45.8)	0.146
	Left	22 (40.7)	11 (36.7)	11 (45.8)	0.687
I-V	Right	3 (5.6)	1 (3.3)	2 (8.3)	0.579
	Left	3 (5.6)	0 (0.0)	3 (12.5)	0.082
WaveV interaural difference[a]	-	6 (11.1)	1 (3.3)	5 (20.8)	0.078
Global Modification	-	48 (88.9)	24 (80.0)	24 (100)	0.028
Variables	Ears	<12 years n (%)	12–18 years n (%)	>18 years n (%)	p
Wave I	Right	0 (0.0)	1 (4.2)	0 (0.0)	0.529
	Left	2 (11.8)	1 (4.2)	0 (0.0)	0.350
Wave III	Right	8 (47.1)	14 (58.3)	4 (30.8)	0.276
	Left	8 (47.1)	13 (54.2)	2 (15.4)	0.068
Wave V	Right	10 (58.8)	17 (70.8)	4 (30.8)	0.062
	Left	8 (47.1)	14 (58.3)	6 (46.2)	0.694
I-III	Right	11 (64.7)	16 (66.7)	3 (23.1)	0.026
	Left	10 (58.8)	20 (83.3)	5 (38.5)	0.020
III-V	Right	3 (17.6)	11 (45.8)	4 (30.8)	0.165
	Left	6 (35.3)	11 (45.8)	5 (38.5)	0.781
I-V	Right	0 (0.0)	2 (8.3)	1 (7.7)	0.480
	Left	0 (0.0)	2 (8.3)	1 (7.7)	0.480
WaveV interaural difference[a]	-	1 (5.9)	4 (16.7)	1 (7.7)	0.503
Global Modification	-	15 (88.2)	24 (100)	9 (69.2)	0.017

n, number; [a] Wave V interaural difference of latency of ≤0.2 ms is considered as normal.

Table 4. Comparison of FFR results between the bilateral ears

Variables	Right Ear	Left Ear	p
	Mean ± SD	Mean ± SD	
Latency V	7.10 ± 0.74	7.37 ± 1.04	0.018
Latency A	8.61 ± 0.95	8.89 ± 1.22	0.065
Latency VA	1.50 ± 0.56	1.52 ± 0.53	0.893
Latency C	18.6 ± 1.00	18.3 ± 1.25	0.269
Latency F	41.1 ± 1.34	41.5 ± 1.75	0.098
Amplitude Va	0.33 (0.25-0.44)	0.35 (0.27-0.46)	0.766
Amplitude Aa	0.19 (0.14-0.31)	0.29 (0.19-0.37)	0.004
Amplitude VAa	0.51 (0.41-0.74)	0.64 (0.48-0.80)	0.139
Amplitude Ca	0.26 (0.16-0.39)	0.29 (0.16-0.43)	0.287
Amplitude Fa	0.26 (0.20-0.40)	0.35 (0.25-0.50)	0.012

SD, standard deviation; a described by median (25-75 percentile).

Table 5. Comparison of the alterations of the FFR results according to sex and age group

Variables	Ears	Total Sample	Female	Male	p
		n (%)	n (%)	n (%)	
Speech-Evoked					
Latency V	Right	20 (37.0)	8 (26.7)	12 (50.0)	0.139
	Left	24 (44.4)	10 (33.3)	14 (58.3)	0.118
Latency A	Right	30 (55.6)	14 (46.7)	16 (66.7)	0.232
	Left	34 (63.0)	15 (50.0)	19 (79.2)	0.055
Latency VA	Right	29 (53.7)	15 (50.0)	14 (58.3)	0.737
	Left	33 (61.1)	18 (60.0)	15 (62.5)	1.000
Latency C	Right	22 (40.7)	10 (33.3)	12 (50.0)	0.337
	Left	17 (31.5)	8 (26.7)	9 (37.5)	0.578
Latency F	Right	26 (48.1)	11 (36.7)	15 (62.5)	0.107
	Left	29 (53.7)	15 (50.0)	14 (58.3)	0.737
Amplitude V	Right	4 (7.4)	2 (6.7)	2 (8.3)	1.000
	Left	3 (5.6)	2 (6.7)	1 (4.2)	1.000
Amplitude A	Right	34 (63.0)	19 (63.3)	15 (62.5)	1.000
	Left	25 (46.3)	16 (53.3)	9 (37.5)	0.376
Amplitude VA	Right	12 (22.2)	6 (20.0)	6 (25.0)	0.913

Table 5. (Continued)

Variables	Ears	Total Sample n (%)	Female n (%)	Male n (%)	p
Amplitude VA	Left	9 (16.7)	5 (16.7)	4 (16.7)	1.000
Amplitude C	Right	18 (33.3)	13 (43.3)	5 (20.8)	0.146
	Left	16 (29.6)	8 (26.7)	8 (33.3)	0.816
Amplitude F	Right	18 (33.3)	9 (30.0)	9 (37.5)	0.771
	Left	10 (18.5)	7 (23.3)	3 (12.5)	0.483
Alteration Conduction	-	53 (98.1)	29 (96.7)	24 (100)	1.000
Variables	Ears	<12 years n (%)	12 – 18 years n (%)	>18 years n (%)	p
Latency V	Right	7 (41.2)	11 (45.8)	2 (15.4)	0.171
	Left	9 (52.9)	13 (54.2)	2 (15.4)	0.053
Latency A	Right	12 (70.6)	12 (50.0)	6 (46.2)	0.313
	Left	13 (76.5)	17 (70.8)	4 (30.8)	0.021
Latency VA	Right	10 (58.8)	12 (50.0)	7 (53.8)	0.856
	Left	13 (76.5)	13 (54.2)	7 (53.8)	0.292
Latency C	Right	8 (47.1)	10 (41.7)	4 (30.8)	0.662
	Left	6 (37.5)	9 (37.5)	1 (7.7)	0.126
Latency F	Right	7 (41.2)	13 (54.2)	6 (46.2)	0.705
	Left	6 (35.3)	15 (62.5)	8 (61.5)	0.184
Amplitude V	Right	1 (5.9)	3 (12.5)	0 (0.0)	0.367
	Left	1 (5.9)	1 (4.2)	1 (7.7)	0.903
Amplitude A	Right	9 (52.9)	14 (58.3)	11 (84.6)	0.168
	Left	9 (52.9)	9 (37.5)	7 (53.8)	0.510
Amplitude VA	Right	4 (23.5)	5 (20.8)	3 (23.1)	0.976
	Left	2 (11.8)	4 (16.7)	3 (23.1)	0.712
Amplitude C	Right	3 (17.6)	9 (37.5)	6 (46.2)	0.220
	Left	7 (41.2)	5 (20.8)	4 (30.8)	0.371
Amplitude F	Right	4 (23.5)	9 (37.5)	5 (38.5)	0.584
	Left	5 (29.4)	4 (16.7)	1 (7.7)	0.301
Alteration Conduction	-	16 (94.1)	24 (100)	13 (100)	0.330

The FFR showed a change in 98.1% of the sample, indicating worse Wave V latency for the left ear, and smaller amplitudes of Wave A and Peak F for the right ear (Table 4). There was no statistically significant difference between the sexes, but the latency of Wave A was later detected in the left ear in the age groups of ≤12 years old and 12 to 18 years old (Table 5).

DISCUSSION

In the present study, the results of electrophysiological evaluation of hearing in patients with SCD were analyzed, and central alterations were revealed through both ABR and FFR.

Reports on the etiology and abnormal findings of ABR have indicated that several diseases may generate similar patterns of response, under condition of effects at the same level of the structure and function of the system [11, 12]. The increase in latencies to the click stimulus can therefore promote a brain stem lesion. [13] In addition, reports have indicated that there is alteration of the central auditory processing associated with the increase of absolute and interpeak latency, and increased latency of the I-III interpeak of the sample indicative of the presence of a low brain stem lesion which is closely associated with auditory processing disorder [14, 15]. These findings may be due to the synaptic delay or delay in neural transmission through incomplete myelination and reduced synaptic efficiency [15].

The FFR is considered an excellent target method to detect central auditory processing disorders [16]. A report has indicated a 85.15% probability of alteration of the central auditory processing in individuals with changes in the FFR [17]. Modification of both the latencies and amplitudes of FFR can be found in the population with altered central auditory processing and language deficits; such findings provide crucial information regarding the generation and propagation of responses along the auditory pathway [16].

The difficulty in perceiving consonants is due to their characteristics of fast and transient low-amplitude signal for speech; whereas, the perception of vowels is more resistant because they constitute a periodic, sustained, and generally higher signal than that of the consonants. Perception of the consonant (transient on set) and vowel (sustained) elicit responses through independent mechanisms [9, 18].

Findings caused by central auditory processing disorder, such as delayed latencies and diminished amplitudes, observed in our study, have also been reported in a previous study [19]. Evaluation through speech provides a more sensitive method to investigate the changes in the synchronicity of response generators and extent of neural allocation represented by the amplitude differences, and rate of transmission of neural impulses during processing represented by the latency differences.

A study has shown significantly increased latencies in the V, A, and C waves of the responses in children with learning disabilities [20]. Another report indicated that the latency deficits through FFR have a negative impact on the processing of acoustic signals in specialized cortical structures for speech [16].

With regard to sex, women tend to have earlier absolute latencies and shorter interpeak intervals than men; this difference is associated with the anatomical inequality of the skull and brain, and size of the cochlea [13, 21, 22, 23]. In our study, this difference was observed in the sample corresponding to male individuals (44.4%).

The delay in the wave for both the ABR and FFR was more significant in the age group of 12 to 18 years-old. In adolescents, the signs and symptoms of the disease alter performance and learning which leads to backwardness in schooling [23, 24]. At the stage of adolescence, many problems arise due to the transition from pediatric treatment to that of the adult and greater avoidance of disease control; [23] these also include death rates of 78.6% in individuals up to 29 years [24]. A study using advanced neuroradiological techniques has reported the occurrence of complications of the central nervous system in 44% and 49% of patients with SCD. A report has indicated that silent ischemic injury associated with several neurocognitive deficits, such as learning problems, attention deficit, lack of executive abilities, poor activity status, and long-term memory [7].

Few studies have focused on the evaluation of ABR in the population with SCD, and none on that of FFR. Ondzotto et al. emphasized the importance of encouraging regular hearing assessment in this population [25]. Further studies are needed to clarify these findings due to the high variability of those between studies; however, the variability may be unavoidable due to the characteristic of SCD itself. Serjeant reported that different geographic areas as well as genetic and environmental factors influence variability in the population with SCD [23].

The analysis of auditory evoked potentials at the level of the brainstem revealed a change in 88.9% of subjects with click stimuli and 98.1% with speech stimulus.

Our overall findings highlight the need for prevention, diagnosis, and systematic follow-up in individuals with SCD, since hearing loss that is undiagnosed or diagnosed late can cause irreparable damage to speech, biopsychosocial, and emotional development.

In conclusion, the changes of the ABR and FFR may be considered as indicators of the individuals' hearing status. The finding of auditory thresholds within the normal range and otoacoustic emissions helps, but does not guarantee excellent sound transmission through the auditory pathway. A new approach as well as further studies focused on central auditory processing and rehabilitation in this population are required. The combined use of electrophysiological assessments such as FFR and behavioral tests of central auditory processing may have effectiveness to clearly guide the possible communicative difficulties and enable earlier and more accurate diagnosis in this population.

REFERENCES

[1] Burch-Sims GP and Matlock VR. 2005. "Hearing loss and auditory function in sickle cell disease." *Journal of Communication Disorders* 38: 321–329. Accessed September 24, 2017. doi: 10.1016/ j.jcomdis. 2005.02.007.

[2] World Health Organization. 2005. "Sickle Cell Anaemia." Report by the secretaria, *Executive Board* 117th session. 5f. 2005.

[3] Ministério da Saúde. Secretaria de Atenção à Saúde. Departamento de Atenção Hospitalar e de Urgência. [Ministry of Health. Secretary of Health Care. Department of Hospital Attention and Emergency]. 2015 *Relatório de Gestão 2013 Coordenação-Geral de Sangue e Hemoderivados* [recurso eletrônico]. Brasília: Ministério da Saúde.

[4] Cançado RD and Jesus JA. 2007. A doença falciforme no Brasil [Sickle cell disease in Brazil]. *Revista Brasileira de Hematologia e Hemoterapia* 29: 203-206. Accessed October 05, 2017 doi: 10.1590/S1516-848420070 00300002.

[5] Hungria H. *Otorrinolaringologia [Otolaryngology]*. Rio de Janeiro: Guanabara Koogan Ltda., 1995).

[6] Silva LP, Nova CV, and Lucena R. 2012. "Sickle cell anemia and hearing loss among children and youngsters: literature review." *Brazilian Journal of Otorhinolaryngology* 78: 126–31.

[7] Ângulo, IL. 2007. "Acidente vascular cerebral e outras complicações do sistema nervoso central nas doenças falciformes." ["Stroke and other complications of the central nervous system in sickle cell disease"]. *Revista Brasileira de Hematologia e Hemoterapia* 29:262-67. Accessed September 18, 2017. doi: 10.1590/S1516-8484200700030 0013.

[8] Intelligent Hearing Systems (IHS). 2017. "Acquiring Click ABR with SmartEP." *Auditory Brainstem Response*, Using Smart EP.

[9] Russo N, Nicol T, Musacchia G, Kraus N. 2004. "Brainstem responses to speech syllables." *Clinical Neurophysiology* 115: 2021-30. Accessed March 20, 2017. doi 10.1016/j.clinph.2004.04.003.

[10] Gonçalves IC. *Aspectos Audiológicos da Gagueira: Evidências Comportamentais e Eletrofisiológicas [Audiological Aspects of Stuttering: Behavioral and Electrophysiological Evidence]*, (Tese (doutorado), Faculdade de Medicina da Universidade de São Paulo, 2013).

[11] Durrant JD and Ferraro JA, Potenciais auditivos evocados de curta latência: eletrococleografia e audiometria de tronco encefálico [Short-latency evoked auditory potentials: electrocochleography and brainstem audiometry], in *Perspectivas Atuais em Avaliação*

Auditiva, ed. Frank E. Musiek and William F. Rintelmann, (Barueri: Manole, 2001), 193-238.

[12] Matas CG and Magliaro FCL, Potencial evocado auditivo de tronco encefálico [Brainstem auditory evoked potential], in *Tratado de Audiologia*, ed. Edilene Boechat (São Paulo: Santos, 2015) 118-112.

[13] Misulis KE. *Manual do Potencial Evocado de Spehlmann: Potenciais Visual, Auditivo e Somatossensitivo Evocados no Diagnóstico Clínico* [*Spehlmann Evoked Potential Manual: Visual, Auditory and Somatosensory Potentials Evoked in Clinical Diagnosis*]. (Rio de Janeiro: Revinter, 2003).

[14] Pfeifer M and Silvana F. 2009. "Auditory processing and auditory brainstem response (ABR)." *CEFAC* 11(suppl 1): 31-37. Accessed in July 23, 2017. http://dx.doi.org/10.1590/S1516-18462009000500006

[15] Rocha-Muniz CN, *Processamento de Sinais Acústicos de Diferentes Complexidades em Crianças com Alteração de Percepção da Audição ou da Linguagem* [*Processing of Acoustic Signs of Different Complexities in Children with Altered Hearing or Language Perception*]. (Tese (Doutorado), Faculdade de Medicina da Universidade de São Paulo, 2011).

[16] Wible B, Nicol T, and Kraus N. 2004. "Atypical brainstem representation of onset and formant structure of speech sounds in children with language-based learning problems." *Biological Psychology* 67: 299–317. Accessed in September 16, 2017. doi: 10.1016/j.biopsycho.2004.02.002.

[17] Rocha-Muniz CN, Filippini R, Neves-Lobo IF, Rabelo CM, Morais AA, Murphy CF, Calarga KS, et al. 2016. "Can speech-evoked auditory brainstem response become a useful tool in clinical practice?" *Codas* 28: 77–80. Accessed July 23, 2017. doi: 10.1590/2317-1782/20162014231.

[18] Abrams DA and Kraus N, "Auditory pathway representations of speech sounds in humans." in *Handbook of Clinical Audiology*, 7th ed. Jack Katz (Philadelphia: Wolters Kluwer, 2015), 527–44.

[19] Filippini R and Schochat E. 2009. "Brainstem evoked auditory potentials with speech stimulus in the auditory processing disorder."

(in English, Portuguese) *Brazilian Journal of Otorhinolaryngology* 75: 449–55. Accessed September 20, 2017.

[20] Kraus N and Nicol T. 2003. "Aggregate neural responses to speech sounds in the central auditory system." *Speech Communication* 41:35–47. Accessed September 16, 2017. doi:10.1016/S0167-6393(02)00091-2.

[21] de Sousa LCA, de Toledo Piza MR, de Freitas Alvarenga K, and Cóser PL, *Eletrofisiologia da Audição e Emissões Otoacústicas: Princípios e Aplicações Clínicas* [*Electrophysiology of Hearing and Otoacoustic Emissions: Principles and Clinical Applications*]. (Ribeirão Preto: Novo Conceito, 2010).

[22] Burkard R and Don M, "Introduction to auditory evoked potentials." in *Handbook of Clinical Audiology*, 7th ed. Jack Katz (Philadelphia: Wolters Kluwer, 2015).

[23] Serjeant GR. 2013. "The natural history of sickle cell disease." *Cold Spring Harbor Perspectives in Medicine* 3(10): a011783. doi: 10.1101/cshperspect.a011783.

[24] Martins GVR, *Adolescente com Doença Falciforme: Conhecimento da Doença e Adesão ao Tratamento* [*Adolescent with Sickle Disease: Knowledge of Disease and Adherence to Treatment*] (Dissertação Mestrado, Universidade Federal do Espírito Santo, Centro de Ciências da Saúde, Vitória, 2015).

[25] Ondzotto G, Malanda F, Galiba J, Ehouo F, Kouassi B, Bamba M. 2002. "Sudden deafness in sickle cell anemia: a case report." (in French) *Bulletin de la Société de pathologie exotique* 95: 248–49.

BIOGRAPHICAL SKETCHES

Adriana Laybauer Silveira

Affiliation: Universidade Federal do Rio Grande do Sul and Hospital de Clínicas de Porto Alegre

Education: Speech Therapist an Audiologist (Instituto Metodista de Educação e Cultura – IMEC), Master Degree in Children and Adolescent Health (Children and Adolescent Health Post Graduate Program, Universidade Federal do Rio Grande do Sul), Doctoral in Children and Adolescent Health (Children and Adolescent Health Post Graduate Program, Universidade Federal do Rio Grande do Sul – in course).

Research and Professional Experience: Research and Audiologist in Hospital de Clínicas de Porto Alegre, RS, Brazil

Link for curriculum vitae: http://lattes.cnpq.br/2630682349601538.

Adriane Ribeiro Teixeira

Affiliation: Universidade Federal do Rio Grande do Sul and Hospital de Clínicas de Porto Alegre

Education: Speech Therapist an Audiologist (Universidade Federal de Santa Maria), Master Degree in Disorders of Human Communication (Universidade Federal de Santa Maria), Doctorate in Biomedical Gerontology (Pontifícia Universidade Católica do Rio Grande do Sul), PhD in Disorders of Human Communication (Universidade Federal de São Paulo)

Research and Professional Experience: Associated Professor of Audiology in Universidade Federal do Rio Grande do Sul, Research and Professor Member of Clinical Staff of Hospital de Clínicas de Porto Alegre

Publications from the Last 3 Years: 23 papers and 110 abstracts on conference proceedings

Link for curriculum: http://lattes.cnpq.br/3147833351413837.

Christina Matzembacher Bittar

Affiliation: Hospital de Clínicas de Porto Alegre

Education: PhD in Medical Sciences, Hematologist

Research and Professional Experience: Hematology Service, Hospital de Clínicas de Porto Alegre (HCPA), Porto Alegre, RS, Brazil

Publications from the Last 3 Years: 1 paper and 10 abstracts on conference proceedings

Link for curriculum: http://lattes.cnpq.br/9363145428906165.

João Ricardo Friedrisch

Affiliation: Hospital de Clínicas de Porto Alegre

Education: PhD in Medical Sciences, Hematologist

Research and Professional Experience: Hematology Service, Hospital de Clínicas de Porto Alegre (HCPA), Porto Alegre, RS, Brazil

Publications from the Last 3 Years: 10 abstracts on conference proceedings

Daniela Pernigotti Dall'Igna

Affiliation: Hospital de Clínicas de Porto Alegre

Education: Graduation in Medicine (Universidade Federal do Rio Grande do Sul), Medical Residence in Otorhinolaryngology (Universidade Federal do Paraná), Specialist in Otorhinolaryngology (Brasilian Society of Otorhinolaryngology).

Research and professional experience:
Research and Otorhinolaryngologist of Hospital de Clínicas de Porto Alegre (RS, Brazil)

Publication from the last 3 years: 30 abstracts on conference proceedings

Link for curriculum: http://lattes.cnpq.br/5470962131607261.

Sergio Saldanha Menna Barreto

Affiliation: Universidade Federal do Rio Grande do Sul

Education: Graduation in Medicine (Universidade Federal de Santa Maria, RS, Brazil), Master Degree in Medicine – Pneumology (Universidade Federal do Rio Grande do Sul, RS, Brazil), Doctorate in Health Science – Cardiology (Universidade Federal do Rio Grande do Sul, RS, Brazil)

Research and professional experience: Professor of Faculty of Medicine in Universidade Federal do Rio Grande do Sul (1978 – 2017)

Publication from the last 3 years: 1 paper and 10 abstracts on conference proceedings

Link for curriculum: http://lattes.cnpq.br/6594237323094386.

INDEX

A

adaptation, 101, 102, 103, 112, 114, 116, 118, 120, 126
adjustment, 101, 102, 107
adults, viii, ix, x, 24, 75, 78, 79, 83, 91, 92, 97, 100, 101, 102, 106, 110, 111, 112, 114
age, x, xi, 20, 24, 27, 30, 34, 37, 57, 59, 100, 101, 103, 105, 107, 108, 109, 110, 111, 131, 142, 143, 145, 146, 147, 149, 150
allele, 6, 8, 9, 10, 12, 13, 14, 32, 70
Alport syndrome, 27, 28, 67, 68
aminoglycosides, 37, 73
amplitude, 145, 149, 150
anxiety, 121, 127
Apert syndrome, 23, 65
array CGH (comparative genomic hybridization), 38, 43, 44, 58
assessment, vii, viii, ix, x, 51, 79, 100, 118, 120, 121, 122, 123, 127, 128, 132, 136, 139, 151
asymmetry, 105, 128, 145
audiograms, 34, 52, 57

audiology, 1, ii, iii, v, 1, 2, 96, 99, 100, 101, 115, 116, 118, 126, 129, 137, 141, 153, 154, 156
auditory evaluation, 143
auditory evoked potentials, 142, 151, 154
auditory performance, 76, 85, 97
auditory stimuli, 134, 139
autosomal dominant, 6, 7, 9, 10, 11, 15, 17, 18, 19, 20, 21, 22, 23, 28, 31, 32, 34, 36, 57, 72
autosomal recessive, vii, viii, 2, 6, 7, 11, 12, 18, 22, 24, 25, 27, 28, 31, 32, 34, 35, 47, 52, 56, 57, 71

B

back pain, 125, 128
backwardness, 150
basilar membrane, 85
benefit, v, vii, viii, ix, x, 50, 51, 53, 54, 58, 81, 85, 99, 100, 101, 102, 103, 104, 105, 106, 107, 108, 111, 112, 113, 114
benefits, ix, 37, 50, 51, 53, 54, 59, 74, 76, 90, 111, 113
benign, 6, 20, 40, 68
benign tumors, 20

bilateral, 20, 21, 24, 27, 106, 111, 143, 145, 147
bioinformatics, 59
biomaterials, 80
biomechanics, 125
blood, 28, 30, 34, 52, 79, 142
blood clot, 34
blood supply, 79
body balance, 118, 120, 123, 130, 131, 132, 134, 135
bone, 38, 85, 86, 87, 89, 94
bone form, 85, 86, 89
bone marrow, 38
brain, 20, 28, 149, 150
brain stem, 149
brainstem, viii, ix, xi, 20, 63, 142, 151, 153, 154
Branchio-oto-renal syndrome, 21, 63, 64
Brazil, viii, ix, xi, 99, 100, 110, 141, 142, 143, 152, 155, 156, 157, 158
breakdown, ix, 76, 87, 91
building blocks, 46

C

candidates, viii, ix, x, 100, 103
cardiac arrest, 27
cardiac arrhythmia, 67
cardiac muscle, 27
cell division, 4, 29, 30, 38
central nervous system, xi, 25, 118, 120, 122, 130, 131, 150, 152
central nervous system (CNS), 131
cerebrospinal fluid, 87
CHARGE syndrome, 18, 19, 61, 62
childhood, 2, 20, 24, 27, 32, 34, 35, 36, 69, 71
children, ix, 7, 8, 9, 10, 11, 14, 16, 17, 22, 25, 51, 55, 60, 63, 64, 67, 68, 75, 77, 78, 79, 80, 88, 90, 91, 92, 96, 126, 131, 136, 138, 150, 152, 154

chorionic villus sampling, 30, 38
chromosome, 5, 6, 13, 14, 15, 26, 29, 30, 37, 38, 40, 41, 42, 72
chromosome 10, 42
chromosomes, 4, 5, 6, 13, 14, 15, 16, 29, 37, 38, 39, 40
cleft palate, 17, 19, 22
clinical application, 50, 127
clinical presentation, 2, 15, 22, 25, 35, 41
cochlea, 31, 36, 80, 81, 82, 83, 84, 85, 86, 87, 89, 94, 96, 131, 143, 150
cochlear implant, vii, viii, ix, 20, 76, 77, 81, 82, 85, 86, 88, 89, 90, 91, 92, 93, 94, 95, 96, 97, 132, 136
cochlear implant failure, 76, 92, 93, 95
complications, 76, 77, 79, 81, 86, 87, 88, 90, 92, 150, 152
conductive hearing loss, 22, 29
configuration, 33, 35, 54, 57
connexin 26, 31, 32, 35, 56, 69
Cornelia de Lange syndrome, 19, 62, 63
correlation, x, xi, 71, 100, 102, 104, 105, 106, 107, 108, 111, 113, 130, 131
correlation coefficient, 105
cross-sectional study, vii, viii, ix, x, 100, 137
Crouzon syndrome, 23, 65
curriculum, 155, 156, 157, 158
cytogenetics, 37, 38, 42, 43
cytomegalovirus, 57, 74

D

datalogging, x, 100, 101, 102, 104, 105, 108, 112, 116
deafness, ix, 2, 6, 7, 8, 9, 10, 12, 14, 18, 24, 35, 37, 52, 56, 59, 60, 66, 67, 69, 70, 71, 72, 73, 74, 75, 126, 137, 155
defects, 18, 19, 27, 29, 33, 36, 65
deletion, 40, 41, 42, 44
depth, 50, 76, 84, 90

Index

diabetes insipidus, 35
diagnostic criteria, 61
disability, 18, 19, 23, 29
disorder, 11, 13, 15, 16, 18, 20, 22, 23, 24, 25, 27, 29, 32, 34, 48, 49, 52, 57, 63, 72, 120, 121, 123, 124, 149, 150, 154
displacement, 21, 82, 87, 93, 133
distribution, 106, 122, 142, 145
DNA (deoxyribonucleic acid), 3, 4, 16, 30, 38, 39, 41, 43, 44, 45, 46, 47, 48, 49, 52, 69, 70
DNA polymerase, 45, 46
DNA repair, 16
DNA sequencing, 48, 70
DNA testing, 38
Down syndrome, 29, 30, 68
duplication, 29, 40, 41, 44

E

education, 101, 103, 106, 108, 109, 111, 112
effusion, 19, 23, 29
elderly, viii, ix, x, 100, 101, 102, 103, 104, 106, 107, 109, 110, 111, 112, 113, 114, 115, 131, 132, 139
electric current, 47
electrical resistance, 88
electrode surface, 96
electrodes, 80, 82, 85, 89
electrophoresis, 46, 47
electrophysiology, 142, 154
end-stage renal disease, 28
environment, 59, 142
environmental factors, 151
etiology, vii, viii, 1, 2, 16, 31, 50, 51, 52, 54, 55, 80, 87, 125, 136, 149
evoked potential, 79, 153
exome sequencing, 2, 48, 49, 50, 57, 58
exposure, 59, 79, 86, 127
extracellular matrix, 35, 65

F

facial asymmetry, 19
facial nerve, 87
facial palsy, 18
families, vii, viii, 2, 6, 23, 26, 50, 51, 52, 53, 54, 55, 56, 57, 66, 68, 70, 71, 72, 73
family history, 20, 51, 52, 53, 56, 57
family members, vii, viii, 2, 7, 28, 52, 54, 55, 57, 104
fibrosis, 82, 84, 86, 87, 89
fibrous tissue, 85, 86, 89, 94
FISH (fluorescence *in situ* hybridization), 38, 41, 42, 44

G

gait, xi, 125, 130, 132, 133
gel electrophoresis, 44, 46, 47
gene expression, 19, 57
genes, 1, 3, 6, 11, 12, 15, 16, 18, 19, 21, 22, 25, 26, 27, 28, 29, 31, 32, 34, 36, 41, 48, 49, 50, 56, 58, 59, 60, 65, 68, 69
genetic background, 65
genetic code, 3
genetic counselling, 70
genetic disease, 142
genetic disorders, 57
genetic syndromes, 29
genetic testing, 2, 11, 37, 50, 51, 52, 53, 54, 55, 56, 58, 59, 67, 74
genetic traits, 7
genetics, v, vii, viii, 1, 2, 5, 23, 37, 42, 44, 47, 50, 51, 52, 53, 54, 58, 60, 64, 66, 67, 68, 69, 73
genome, 4, 15, 16, 36, 37, 44, 48, 49, 50, 57
genotype, 6, 12, 17, 47, 66, 71
growth, 18, 19, 20, 38, 77, 80, 89, 96, 140

H

hair, 23, 33, 34, 70, 71, 85
hair cells, 33, 34, 70, 85
Handicap Inventory for the Elderly - Screening Version, 102
health, 50, 53, 54, 55, 58, 60, 110, 112, 115, 116
health care, 50, 55, 58, 110
health effects, 50
health problems, 58
health services, 115
hearing, v, vii, viii, ix, x, xi, 1, 2, 3, 7, 9, 11, 17, 18, 19, 20, 21, 22, 23, 24, 25, 27, 28, 29, 31, 32, 33, 34, 35, 36, 37, 50, 51, 52, 53, 54, 55, 56, 57, 58, 59, 60, 61, 63, 64, 66, 67, 68, 69, 70, 71, 72, 73, 74, 77, 79, 89, 91, 93, 99, 100, 101, 102, 103, 104, 105, 106, 107, 108, 109, 110, 111, 112, 113, 114, 115, 116, 120, 125, 126, 130, 132, 134, 135, 136, 137, 138, 142, 143, 144, 149, 151, 152, 153, 154
hearing aid, v, viii, ix, x, 99, 100, 101, 102, 103, 104, 105, 106, 107, 108, 109, 111, 112, 113, 114, 115, 116, 132, 137, 138
Hearing Handicap Inventory for Adults, x, 100, 102
hearing impairment, xi, 66, 69, 73, 102, 130, 132, 135
hearing loss, v, vii, viii, ix, x, xi, 1, 2, 3, 7, 9, 11, 17, 18, 19, 20, 21, 22, 23, 24, 25, 27, 28, 29, 31, 32, 33, 34, 35, 36, 37, 50, 51, 52, 53, 54, 55, 56, 57, 58, 59, 60, 63, 64, 67, 68, 69, 70, 71, 72, 73, 100, 101, 102, 103, 104, 105, 106, 107, 108, 109, 110,111, 114, 116, 120, 125, 126, 130, 132, 134, 136, 137, 138, 143, 151, 152
hearing loss counseling, 2
hemoglobinopathy, viii, ix, xi, 142, 143
history, 27, 51, 53, 56, 57, 120, 138, 154
human, viii, ix, xi, 3, 4, 5, 16, 38, 42, 44, 48, 49, 60, 62, 63, 70, 71, 72, 73, 93, 94, 106, 118, 119, 121, 130, 131
human body, xi, 4, 119, 130
human development, 62
human genome, 3, 4, 5, 44, 48, 49, 60
human subjects, 94

I

identification, 26, 50, 59, 120
impaired, 101
implant failures, 92, 93, 95
implants, 63, 82, 86, 90, 93
in situ hybridization, 41, 42
incidence, 17, 18, 19, 20, 22, 23, 24, 27, 57, 85, 143
individuals, xi, 9, 21, 22, 24, 25, 29, 32, 36, 37, 54, 59, 77, 111, 115, 142, 145, 149, 150, 151
infection, 2, 57, 77, 79, 83
inflammatory mediators, 86
inflammatory responses, 80
inheritance, vii, viii, 2, 6, 8, 9, 10, 11, 12, 13, 14, 16, 17, 22, 23, 28, 31, 56, 57, 64
injury prevention, 127, 140
inner ear, 18, 21, 24, 27, 76, 81, 131
insertion, 76, 80, 81, 82, 84, 85, 87, 89, 90
integrity, 77, 81, 83
intensive care unit, 127, 138
intervention, 74, 124, 135
isolation, 1, 3, 26, 31, 134
issues, 27, 53, 55, 103, 112

J

Jacobsen syndrome, 34
Jervell and Lange-Nielsen syndrome, 27, 53, 67

Index

K

karyotype, 5, 6, 38, 40, 42, 43, 44
karyotyping, 38, 39, 41, 44
kidney, 18, 21, 27, 52
kidney transplantation, 28

L

latency, 145, 146, 148, 149, 150, 153
learning disabilities, 150
level of education, 104
Louisiana, 1, 5, 24, 25, 42, 47, 67

M

magnet, 82, 83, 87, 93
magnetic resonance, 82
magnetic resonance imaging, 82
management, 67, 68, 72, 96, 125, 128, 136
measurement, 122, 132, 145
median, 105, 106, 107, 108, 147
medical, 18, 50, 54, 57, 95, 145
medicine, 44, 118, 127, 130, 154
MELAS, 28, 68
MERRF, 28, 68
meta-analysis, 69, 137, 140
microscope, 39, 40, 41
mitochondria, 15, 17, 28, 36, 37
mitochondrial, 6, 9, 15, 16, 17, 28, 31, 36, 68, 73
molecular biology, 44
morphology, 38, 110
mosaicism, 29, 40
muscles, 28, 125, 131
musculoskeletal, 126
mutations, 6, 11, 16, 18, 19, 20, 21, 22, 23, 24, 26, 27, 28, 31, 32, 33, 34, 35, 36, 38, 49, 56, 61, 62, 63, 64, 66, 68, 69, 70, 71, 72, 73

N

negative consequences, 59
nerve, 18, 20, 87, 131
nervous system, 20, 28, 118, 131
neurofibromatosis type 1, 20
neurofibromatosis type 2, 20, 63
neuropathy, 33, 57, 70
nondisjunction, 29, 30, 40
nonsyndromic hearing loss, 1, 2, 24, 31, 33, 34, 36, 50, 52, 56, 57, 70, 72
nuclear genome, 16, 36
nucleic acid, 3, 4
nucleotides, 3, 46
nucleus, 4, 15, 16, 92

O

occupational therapy, 124
operations, 86, 87, 120
optic glioma, 20
organ, 131, 132
organelles, 15, 16
organism, 142
organs, xi, 118, 119, 122, 123, 130, 131, 142
ossification, 80, 81, 84, 86, 89
otitis media, 19, 23, 29
otoacoustic emissions, xii, 142, 151
Outcome Inventory for Hearing Aids (IOI-HA), x, 100, 102, 104, 105, 106, 107, 108, 109, 111, 113, 115
outpatient, viii, ix, xi, 82, 104, 105, 142, 143

P

parallelism, 122
parents, 7, 10, 11, 12, 19, 22, 51, 54, 55
participants, 106, 111, 112, 143

patient care, vii, viii, 2
patterns of inheritance, 6
Pendred syndrome, 24, 33, 66
penetrance, 9, 11, 22, 65
peripheral blood, 38
permission, iv, 5, 42, 47
phenotype, 6, 61, 66, 68, 71
physical activity, 121, 124, 135
physical features, 17, 21, 23, 29
platform, xi, 118, 122, 130, 132, 139
polymerase, 41, 44, 45
polymerase chain reaction, 41, 44, 46
polymorphisms, 6, 59, 71
population, ix, 25, 26, 31, 59, 76, 77, 80, 85, 100, 110, 111, 114, 116, 142, 143, 149, 150, 151
positive correlation, x, xi, 100
postural control, xi, 118, 123, 125, 127, 130, 131, 132, 136, 137
posture, vi, viii, ix, xi, 118, 119, 120, 121, 123, 124, 125, 126, 127, 128, 129, 130, 131, 135, 136, 137
preparation, iv, 38, 39, 74
preservation, ix, 76, 89
preterm infants, 127, 138
prevention, 67, 101, 135, 139, 140, 151
principles, 41, 74, 143
proteins, 3, 4, 18, 19, 21, 26, 29, 31, 33, 39, 49, 63, 70, 142
psychometric properties, 115

Q

quality of life, 101, 132, 143
questionnaire, x, xi, 100, 102, 104, 105, 106, 108, 111, 112, 113

R

receptors, 118, 119, 120, 122, 123, 124, 132
recognition, vii, viii, ix, 76, 90, 91, 94, 111

recurrence, vii, viii, 2, 11, 13, 23, 53, 54
rehabilitation, xi, 64, 88, 91, 101, 115, 118, 130, 132, 138, 151
reliability, ix, 76, 94, 125
response, viii, ix, xi, 79, 86, 105, 118, 120, 142, 149, 150, 153, 154
restriction in social participation, v, vii, viii, ix, x, 99, 100, 101, 102, 104, 105, 106, 107, 108, 111, 112, 113
restrictions, 101, 103, 105, 111
retinitis pigmentosa, 24, 25
Rett syndrome, 15
revision surgery, v, vii, viii, ix, 75, 76, 80, 84, 87, 91, 97
risk, xi, 10, 12, 14, 17, 27, 29, 30, 36, 40, 52, 54, 76, 82, 83, 84, 87, 130, 132, 134, 136, 139
risk assessment, 36
risk factors, 139

S

satisfaction, v, vii, viii, ix, x, 99, 100, 101, 102, 103, 104, 105, 106, 107, 108, 111, 112, 113, 114, 115, 116
schooling, 111, 150
science, 59, 65, 118
self-assessment, 102, 114
self-reports, 103, 111, 112
sensorineural hearing loss, 21, 24, 25, 27, 33, 35, 52, 60, 69, 73, 126, 137
sensory system, 131
sex, x, xi, 5, 6, 12, 29, 38, 100, 105, 106, 108, 110, 111, 146, 147, 150
sickle cell, 142, 151, 152, 154, 155
sickle cell anemia, 155
sickle cell disease, vi, viii, ix, xi, 141, 142, 151, 152, 154
signs, 11, 16, 19, 20, 21, 22, 27, 79, 150
skewed X-inactivation, 15

Index

skin, 20, 21, 23, 36, 38, 52, 73, 79, 83, 87, 119, 125
skin diseases, 73
social participation, vii, viii, ix, x, 100, 101, 102, 103, 104, 105, 106, 107, 108, 111, 112, 113, 116
software, x, xi, 43, 44, 59, 88, 89, 100, 108
speech, vii, viii, ix, 76, 77, 78, 79, 80, 88, 90, 91, 94, 101, 102, 103, 111, 143, 149, 150, 151, 152, 154
speech perception, 77, 79, 80, 90
speech sounds, 154
stability, 45, 118, 119, 123, 125, 126, 128, 135, 136, 137, 139
standard deviation, 105, 107, 108, 145, 147
Stickler syndrome, 17, 18, 61
stimulation, 77, 79, 85, 89, 96, 123, 124, 128, 134
stimulus, 79, 145, 149, 151, 154
structural defects, 21
structure, 3, 4, 15, 21, 33, 37, 149, 154
surgical outcome, v, 76, 85
surgical technique, 95
surgical techniques, 95
symptoms, 16, 73, 78, 79, 81, 101, 143, 150
syndrome, 15, 16, 17, 18, 19, 21, 22, 23, 24, 25, 26, 27, 28, 29, 30, 33, 34, 35, 42, 47, 50, 52, 53, 54, 58, 61, 62, 63, 64, 65, 66, 67, 68, 70, 72, 126
syndromic hearing loss, 2, 16, 17, 53, 56, 73

T

techniques, 2, 41, 48, 58, 89, 150
temperature, 41, 45, 46, 70
testing, 2, 30, 37, 38, 42, 44, 48, 49, 50, 51, 53, 54, 55, 56, 57, 58, 59, 79, 81, 84, 116
three-dimensional reconstruction, 86
tinnitus, 20, 35, 78, 120, 125, 132, 135, 137, 139
tissue, 38, 84, 85, 86

tonic, xi, 118, 119, 120, 122, 130, 132
training, 125, 127, 139
translocation, 40, 44, 81, 82
transmission, 8, 149, 150, 151
trauma, ix, 76, 82, 83, 85, 86, 87, 120, 126
Treacher Collins syndrome, 22, 65
treatment, ix, 53, 54, 65, 72, 75, 79, 124, 126, 138, 150
tympanometry, xi, 142, 144

U

Usher syndrome, 24, 25, 26, 33, 47, 53, 66, 67, 70

V

variable expressivity, 22
vertigo, 20, 87, 121, 124, 126, 132, 137
vestibular disorders, viii, ix, xi, 128, 130, 132, 134, 135, 138
vestibular schwannoma, 20
vestibular system, xi, 81, 118, 119, 130, 132
vestibulocochlear nerve, 20
vision, 18, 20, 23, 24, 27, 35, 52, 53, 125

W

Waardenburg syndrome, 21, 22, 64
whole genome sequencing, 48, 49
Wolfram syndrome, 35, 72

X

X chromosome, 5, 6, 8, 12, 14, 15
X-inactivation, 8, 15
X-linked, 6, 8, 12, 14, 15, 20, 27, 28, 31, 36, 73

Y

Y chromosome, 6, 14, 29

The Role of Communication Partners in the Audiological Rehabilitation

AUTHORS: Vinaya Manchaiah, Ph.D. and Brian Taylor

SERIES: Audiology and Hearing Research Advances

BOOK DESCRIPTION: *The Role of Communication Partners in the Audiological Rehabilitation* uncovers the psychological and social processes that the communication partners of persons with hearing loss may experience. Currently, there is a renewed focus on family-centered audiological rehabilitation.

SOFTCOVER ISBN: 978-1-53612-817-8
RETAIL PRICE: $160

Sensorineural Hearing Loss: Prevalence, Risk Factors and Treatment

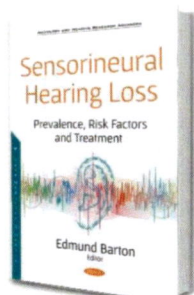

EDITOR: Edmund Barton

SERIES: Audiology and Hearing Research Advances

BOOK DESCRIPTION: Sensorineural hearing loss, if not properly treated, may likely compromise speech and, consequently, the psychosocial development of the affected child. Therefore, early diagnosis and treatment has a significant impact on the likelihood of hearing rehabilitation and on social development. The authors provide an analysis of the prevalence, stratification of risk factors, and the most appropriate treatment for sensorineural hearing loss.

SOFTCOVER ISBN: 978-1-53614-475-8
RETAIL PRICE: $82

Advances in Hearing Healthcare Informatics: The Measurement of Speech Recognition Ability in an Aging Population

Authors: Wayne M. Garrison, Ph.D. and Joseph H. Bochner, Ph.D.

Series: Audiology and Hearing Research Advances

Book Description: This publication details the development of a hearing screening application that is: (1) Self-administering; (2) Can be taken in the privacy of one's home; (3) Short in duration; and (4) Freely available for use. The application is shown to serve as a proxy for pure-tone hearing screening methods, using the criteria established by the American Speech-Language-Hearing Association (ASHA).

Hardcover ISBN: 978-1-53614-361-4
Retail Price: $160

Cochlear Implants: Advances, Efficacy and Future

Editor: Herbert W. Courtney

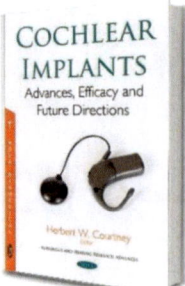

Series: Audiology and Hearing Research Advances

Book Description: *Cochlear Implants: Advances, Efficacy and Future Directions* assesses the growing need to provide other measures for assessing the impact of cochlear implantation. As such, this book aims to evaluate the Cross-Modal Plasticity in deaf children with visual-impairment after CI use, through the analysis of changes in the topographic distribution of the cortical response of Somatosensory Evoked Potential by stimulation of the median nerve.

Softcover ISBN: 978-1-53613-208-3
Retail Price: $82